PENGUIN BOOKS

P9-EEA-368

THE DEATH OF PSYCHIATRY

E. Fuller Torrey was graduated magna cum laude from Princeton University and took his M.A. in anthropology at Stanford and his M.D. at McGill. He has taught at the Albert Einstein College of Medicine and, as an administrative and research psychiatrist, is now Special Assistant to the Director of International Activities at the National Institute of Mental Health. Dr. Torrey is also the author of *The Mind Game: Witchdoctors and Psychiatrists*. He lives in Washington, D.C.

E. FULLER TORREY, M.D.

The Death of Psychiatry

Penguin Books Inc
New York • Baltimore

Penguin Books Inc
72 Fifth Avenue
New York, New York 10011

Penguin Books Inc
7110 Ambassador Road
Baltimore, Maryland 21207

Penguin Books Canada Limited
41 Steelcase Road West
Markham, Ontario, Canada L3R 1B4

First published by Chilton Book Company,
    Radnor, Pennsylvania, 1974
Published by Penguin Books Inc, 1975

Copyright © E. Fuller Torrey, 1974

Printed in the United States of America

RC
455.2
M4 T69   /   22,515

*The opinions set forth in this volume are those of
the author and do not represent the official policy
of the National Institute of Mental Health or
the United States Public Health Service.*

CAMROSE LUTHERAN COLLEGE
LIBRARY

To BILL *and* NANCY SCOONES
for Their Friendship

Preface

PSYCHIATRY is an emperor standing naked in his new clothes. It has worked and striven for 70 years to become an emperor, a full brother with the other medical specialties. And now it stands there resplendent in its finery. But it does not have any clothes on; and even worse, nobody has told it so. To tell an emperor that he does not have any clothes on has never been advocated as the best way to win friends. The alternative, however, is equally painful, for you must then become part of the general delusion. Each of us must choose our own way out of this dilemma.

This book is both an attack upon the medical model of psychiatry and a proposal for an alternative model. As an attack, it is certainly not the first, nor will it be the last. Criticism of the medical model has come from within the psychiatric profession and from without. Szasz, Laing, Fouchault, Liefer, Coles, Albee, Fromm, Ryan, Sarbin, Sheff, Goffman, and many others have attacked it, though not all for the same reasons.

Occasionally such attacks imply that the medical model has been purposefully perpetrated on an unsuspecting public by psychiatrists as a means of repression or social control. Such allegations I explicitly disavow. The medical model was an honest and humanitarian attempt to solve the problems of deviant human behavior. That it has not turned out to be a very good solution should not detract from its original intent. Allegations of a conspiracy also have the shortcoming of implying a plan; anyone who has seen American psychiatry in action knows that no planning of any kind takes place so that a conspiracy would be impossible.

The book is divided into two parts. The first part is a catalogue of the absurd endpoints of the medical model of psychiatry. Chapter 1 provides a framework within which to view the death of psychiatry. Chapter 2 puts the medical model in historical perspective and shows how we got where we are. Chapter 3 examines the current scene, focusing on systems of "psychotherapy" to demonstrate how thin the medical veneer really is. Chapters 4 through 7 examine the underpinnings of the medical structure, showing that conceptually and semantically the foundations are built upon sand. Moreover, the structure itself is deficient, with uprights infested by termites and a roof that is falling in. The argument in most cases is deductive from the theory to the practice. In all cases, it is shown that psychiatry, as the medical model of deviant human behavior, is dysfunctional.

The second part of the book then develops an alternative model of human behavior, basically educational in design. Chapter 8 examines the contemporary educational scene and shows how, in its present form, it cannot serve as a model even for itself. Chapter 9 discusses behavioral science and tutors, two concepts badly needed by education which have been sequestered off in other corners. Chapter 10 considers a series of twenty-eight individuals who are currently called "psychiatric patients" and asks the question: Do these people have brain disease or do they have problems of living? Chapters 11 through 13 spell out the dimensions and ramifications of a neo-educational model in greater detail and attempt to show how such a model solves the problems left unsolved by the medical model. Finally, Chapter 14 reviews the difficulties which are likely to be encountered as psychiatry dies and a model such as the neo-educational one takes its place.

I have drawn heavily on many people's ideas and am not certain whether I am really an author or an editor. Wherever I can remember, I have indicated my debt specifically. There are other places, however, where my debt is to a composite of the whole bibliography. I also owe much to those who read portions of the manuscript, especially Nancy and Bill Scoones, Ann and Bob Taylor, Linda Hess, and Harold Wise. And to my wife Barbara, I owe ultimately all my ideas of merit.

Contents

Part I
The Medical Model

After forty-one years of medical activity, my self-knowledge tells me that I have never really been a doctor in the proper sense. I became a doctor through being compelled to deviate from my original purpose; and the triumph of my life lies in my having, after a long and roundabout journey, found my way back to my earliest path.

SIGMUND FREUD
Postscript to a Discussion on Lay Analysts

1

An Irish Wake for Psychiatry

PSYCHIATRY is dying. This seems ironic in view of the fact that more people than ever are going to more psychiatrists than ever. But it is dying nevertheless, slowly being suffocated by the stethoscope which it has worn around its neck. And its demise is going largely unheralded. This hardly seems fair; psychiatry has made many contributions to our civilization during its lifetime and it should be properly recognized.

What psychiatry really deserves is an Irish wake. Such an event would appropriately express both the sorrow we feel at its passing and the pride we feel at having known it and been part of it. In its three score and ten years, psychiatry has lived a full and productive life. It has not only elevated the study of human behavior to the level of respectability, but has removed it once and for all from the realm of theology. The demons thought to be possessing the mentally "ill" have finally been put to rest. Psychiatry, moreover, has provided many people who have problems of living with well trained "therapists" to whom they can go for help in solving personal problems.

At the same time, an Irish wake would make it clear to everyone that we recognize the fact of psychiatry's death. Like all deaths, we find it easier to deny than to accept. And when the death is that of a social and cultural institution like psychiatry, it is that much more difficult to accept. We are a sentimental people who treasure our past. And our culture values only enlargement and birth; it has not yet learned how to equally value diminution and death.

In the case of an institution like psychiatry, our inability to let it die gracefully becomes a serious matter. We insist that it continue to do a job which it is no longer capable of doing. The consequence is that the job gets done very poorly, or it doesn't get done at all. We try to deny it but denials are in vain—once an institution has lived its allotted time, it will die whether we want it to or not.

A useful approach to understanding what is currently happening to psychiatry is that of Thomas Kuhn, a philosopher of science. In *The Structure of Scientific Revolutions,* Kuhn shows that advancements in science are related to changes in paradigms or models. A paradigm or model, used in this sense, is a shared system of assumptions and rules of conduct for a scientific endeavor. The Copernican model of the earth moving around the sun (rather than the opposite) is an example. Drawing upon historical changes in physics, astronomy, and other sciences for examples, Kuhn details how change begins when anomalies are noted in the existing model. The anomalies increase until there is a general sense of malfunction of the model. This precipitates crises as the old model is bent, trying to make it accommodate data that no longer fit. The next step is a search for new models which will fit; a search which is ultimately resolved by determining which new model functions best.

This is what is occurring in psychiatry. The medical model is equivalent to the model of the sun revolving around the earth. More and more anomalies are being perceived and we are furiously bending the medical model to try and make it accommodate them. But the data are square and the holes are round. A general sense of malfunction is emerging, creating crises and the beginnings of a search for new models.

Only recently have we been able to perceive the malfunctions of the medical model. For many years, psychiatry fought furiously for acceptance as a medical specialty. During the battle, a quiet and dispassionate analysis was not possible. Now that psychiatry has won its place within medicine, the medical model can be carried through to its logical conclusions. The product is chaos. It is as if psychiatry had been represented as a late, unwanted daughter of Asclepius who was being denied her birthright; after years of fighting for it, she is finally accepted, only to then realize that she isn't really Asclepius' child after all.

Psychiatry, then, is ultimately dying because it can now be seen as nonfunctional. As a medical model approach to problems of human behavior, it produces confusions rather than solutions. If we are wise, we will allow it to die with dignity and not try to prop it up to do a job it is no longer able to do. Its death is not necessarily a negative event, for it makes possible the birth of a true behavioral science. The latter cannot come into existence as long as psychiatry lingers on.

In keeping with Kuhn, then, the death of psychiatry is seen as a single event on an evolutionary scale whereby all our institutions and ideas evolve. This is very difficult for us to comprehend, however. When we have grown up assuming that the sun revolves around the earth, it is very difficult for us to think of it any other way. We *know* that it is true, just as we *know* that the study of certain kinds of human behavior should be part of medicine. We can reevaluate single facts in our minds, but to ask us to reevaluate whole models seems like too great a task. It should be noted that even in the field of human behavior, however, there is precedent for doctors supporting some very mistaken models. Doctors, for instance, played an important role in the Massachusetts witchcraft trials, introducing important "scientific" evidence which "proved" the guilt of the accused as "witches."[2] What gives us the right now as psychiatrists to assume that we are not just as mistaken about the medical model? That is why I would say, with Kuhn, that "my most fundamental objective is to urge a change in the perception and evaluation of familiar data."

2

An Historical Perspective: Origins of the Medical Model

PSYCHIATRY as we know it did not, like Minerva, spring fully grown from the head of Jupiter. Rather it is the logical outgrowth of historical trends which culminated, late in the nineteenth century, in the categorization of irrational behavior under the medical model as "disease." At the time, that categorization appeared to be both logical and correct. From the vantage point of the present, however, we can see that it was a mistake.

It is not easy to examine the history of psychiatry in an objective way. Most of the accounts are written by physicians with the assumption of the medical model as "truth." The history is chosen and synthesized to show how everything leads up to the contemporary physician-psychiatrist, "treating" irrational behavior as mental "illness." In order to do this, the physician-authors often have to bend facts beyond credibility; but even after all their efforts, the facts remain embarrassingly unmalleable.

A good example is Gregory Zilboorg's *History of Medical Psychology.* Like most psychiatrists, Zilboorg sees the history of irrational behavior as an inexorable trek toward the meccas of medical psychiatry:

> Psychiatry, almost from the moment it was delivered from the womb of medicine in the days of Hippocrates, was kidnapped and brought up in the strange home of theology and in the flowery, multi-colored gardens of abstract philosophy.

Zilboorg then tries to justify, in over 500 pages, his assumption that medicine was indeed the mother. In the end, however, he seems disquieted about what he has turned up.

> One of the most conspicuous features of psychiatric history is that it is totally different from medical history. Psychiatry still lags behind medicine as to the certainty of its task, the sphere of its activity, and the methods to be pursued. General medicine, in the narrow sense of the word, never had to ask itself what disease is. It always knew what it meant to be ill, for both the patient and the doctor knew what pain and other forms of physical suffering were. Psychiatry never had such a clear criteria of illness. Only a very small proportion of the mentally ill show any suffering: very few if any are aware that their suffering is caused by a mental illness.... Medicine had less differences with the medieval barbers who practiced surgery than it has today with psychiatry. The history of twenty-four centuries of medicine shows clearly that there has always been a strong and deep-seated antagonism between medicine and psychiatry.[2]

What happens when the history of irrational behavior is reviewed without assuming a medical model as truth? First we see the explanations for such behavior being channeled into three broad streams—the religious, the medical, and the psychological. The first two are older and wider; the third newer, narrower, but more rapid. The first two fuse at their source, as in the physician-priests of Mesopotamia, and have run quietly parallel or tried to dominate the other at different periods over the centuries. The medical stream finally prevailed permanently in the nineteenth century and then went on to absorb the smaller and newer stream of psychology.

The medical stream dates back at least to the Greek theories of humors. Irrational behavior of various kinds was attributed to an imbalance of the humors—depression, for instance, was due to excessive bile. Another medical explanation was that of a displaced organ, as in explaining hysteria by a wandering uterus. These were the early beginnings of the medical model that has come to dominate our thinking about irrational behavior; the idea that "for every distorted thought there is a distorted molecule" is just a more sophisticated extension of this model. The person behaving irrationally is "sick" just as surely as a gallstone causes pain.

Simultaneously, the religious stream was being used to explain irrational behavior. People were thought to act irrationally because they were possessed by devils or demons. During the Middle Ages, this stream became dominant and maintained its ascendancy for over 1,000 years. It reached its culmination in the witch-hunts, staunchly supported by the church. Pope Innocent VIII issued a papal bull in 1484 in support of witch-hunting; and two Jesuit theologians wrote the notorious *Malleus Maleficarum,* the bird book of witch-hunting which not only tells you how to recognize various witches by their color, call, and behavior, but also prescribes the best torture to confirm identification in each case. The Greek idea that people acting irrationally were "sick" was supplanted by the theological idea that they were "possessed." The religious stream received further reinforcement from the control of leprosy in the late Middle Ages; another moral scapegoat was needed to take the place of the leper and "madmen" possessed by devils offered a suitable substitute.[3]

From the early Renaissance onward, the medical stream slowly regained dominance as an explanation of irrational behavior. At Geel, Belgium, the word "sickroom" was written over the annex to the church where "possessed" people were coming to be "cured" in the thirteenth century.[4] A major step was the beginning of confinement for such persons. Although at first this was done just as part of a general confinement of the poor and criminal, it soon developed a medical rationale. The ships of fools came to anchor and they were called "hospitals." From the end of the eighteenth century, the medical certificate became almost obligatory for the confinement of madmen.[5] Simultaneously, religious explanations of irrational behavior ebbed.

THE ERA OF THE MISTAKE

We move now into the nineteenth century, the era of the mistake. This is the century when the psychological stream emerged to challenge the medical and religious streams, only to be absorbed by the former when the challenge was barely uttered.

The first striking fact to notice about this era is that medicine had never been stronger. This is the century of rationalism and positivism, the belief that man was governed by natural laws and that all these laws could be elucidated through science. It was the era of Darwin showing man in his place alongside other species, fixed there by laws of natural selection. Freud himself acknowledged a strong attraction to Darwin's theories, "...for they held out hopes of an extraordinary advance in our understanding of the world."[6]

In medicine, the major advances were in microbiology and surgery, both reinforcing the role of the patient as a passive receptacle for organisms, stones, and growths. Virchow, Pasteur, Lister, and Semmelweis in the 1850s and 1860s began the trend. Then when Koch demonstrated the bacteria that causes anthrax in 1876, a period began which was to bring new discoveries of bacteria and other organisms almost monthly for the next 25 years. There was every reason to believe that bacteria would explain everything wrong with man, including his occasionally irrational behavior. Further support for such thoughts came from the three most common nonsurgical diseases of the era—syphilis, tuberculosis, and typhoid. Each sometimes produced irrational thinking or behavior in those it afflicted; other such thinking or behavior, it was reasoned, must be caused by other diseases.

The rise of neurology in this era further reinforced the medical model. For the first time, it began to be possible not just to speculate about brain diseases but to actively explore them. Sir Charles Bell initiated the neurological advances in 1811 with his proposal about how sensations are carried by the spinal cord. Neurophysiology received an impetus from the work of Hitzig and Fritsch in the 1860s, electrically stimulating the brains of dogs and later of people. Sechenov and Pavlov carried on this mechanistic tradition and further refined the idea that the brain was a stimulus-response machine. Advances in neuroanatomy resulted in localization of specific areas of the brain for specific function (e.g., speech). Studies in neurohistology clarified the cell structure of the brain and brought Golgi and Ramon y Cajal a Nobel Prize in 1906. The status of eminent neurologists was very high—men like Carl Wernicke in Germany, John Hughlings Jackson in England, and Silas Weir Mitchell in America—and all believed that irrational behavior was caused by mental "disease," disease in the brain.

In the midst of these advances in microbiology and neurology, psychiatry began to emerge as an entity. And it was firmly a medical entity. Its province was restricted to only a portion of people who were acting irrationally—the insane, madmen, and lunatics. Most of these people we now call "psychotics." The leaders of this emerging medical specialty were Griesinger in Germany, Maudsley in England, and Rush in the United States; and all were strongly medically inclined. Psychological explanations of irrational behavior were anathema to them. Griesinger believed that "we recognize in every case of mental disease a morbid action of that organ [the brain].'" And Rush, the founder of American psychiatry, used a spinning chair as his main therapeutic tool to counteract congested blood in the brain:

> In my intended publication upon madness, I hope to satisfy you that the disease is arterial, and that without morbid action in the blood vessels of the brain no form of the disease can exist.[8]

Virtually all of these early psychiatrists agreed that masturbation, because of its adverse effects on the human body, was a major cause of insanity.

This total medicalization of irrational behavior culminated with Emil Kraepelin. In the early years of the twentieth century, he put the final medical seal on irrational behavior by naming it and categorizing it. Irrational behavior could now hold its head up in medical company for it had names— names like dementia praecox and paranoia. These names described everything and explained nothing. Kraepelin believed strongly that irrational behavior was caused by heredity and constitution. He was antipsychological and a therapeutic nihilist. His classificatory system continues to dominate psychiatry up to the present, not because it has proven of value—indeed it is largely ignored by younger psychiatrists—but because it has been the ticket of admission for irrational behavior into medicine.

THE PSYCHOLOGICAL STREAM

It was into this pool of rationalism and positivism, of microbiology and neurology, that the psychological stream tried to come into its own. No wonder that it failed and was almost immediately swallowed up by medicine.

But the psychological stream is not really part of medicine nor has it ever been. It differed fundamentally from both the medical and religious streams dominant up to that point because it fixed the cause of irrational behavior as being within the control of the individual. Medicine and religion had fixed the control elsewhere—in devils or in disordered brain cells. But the psychological view looked to man. Franz Alexander aptly sums up the difficulty in arriving at this view historically:

> It appears, indeed, that man has a deep disinclination to understand the disturbances of his behavior in terms of psychology. He undoubtedly shuns the responsibility which results from such understanding and is ready to blame the spirits, the devil, or even mystical fluids in his body for abnormal behavior instead of recognizing that it is the result of his own feelings, strivings, and inner conflicts.[9]

The psychological stream did not arise *de nouveau* in the nineteenth century. Its roots stretched back into the Greek tradition of rational psychology, the belief that reason will enable a person to overcome error and irrational behavior. New behavior, in this system, was thought to be brought about by admonitions and exhortations. Through the ages, small contributions to the psychological stream continued to appear, but they were always overshadowed by the other dominant traditions. Johann Weyer, sixteenth century physician, advocated seeing witches as "poor, miserable, old, deteriorated, and melancholic women" rather than as possessed by demons. He even used techniques similar to modern "psychotherapy."[10] But his contribution is so unusual that it simply provides a relief against which to observe the dominant picture of that period.

Another contribution to this stream was the work of Pinel and Tuke. Through their emphasis on the humanness of "madmen," they focused on the person himself. When they cut the chains and freed "the insane," they were not only liberating them so that medicine could claim them as "patients," but also allowing irrational behavior to be seen as human action by human beings. This was an important precedent for psychology.

Franz Mesmer, the father of hypnotism, was another contributor to the psychological stream. He believed that his powers were due to a magnetic fluid, so he was actually in the mechanistic-medical tradition. However, the net effect of his contribution was to advance the psychological approach considerably. He was the first to appreciate the qualities of the person doing the "magnetizing." By the nineteenth century, textbooks on magnetism included a chapter on the personality of the magnetizer and his professional ethics.[11] Nor did Mesmer believe it was necessary to be a physician to be a good magnetizer. The golden age of magnetism in the first half of the nineteenth century produced a dual concept of conscious and unconscious, exploration of the psychological dimensions of the mind, and the realization that one person could help another to change his irrational behavior.

Magnetism exerted a powerful influence on the thought and literature of the nineteenth century. Schopenhauer said that "from a philosophical point of view, Animal Magnetism is the most momentous discovery ever made."[12] Others like Poe and Balzac were similarly influenced. And it was from the writers and philosophers of the period that the psychological stream received its greatest impetus. Nietzsche, Herbart, Fechner, Stendhal, Shaw, and Ibsen all wrote insightful accounts of human motivations and behavior. Dostoevsky's brilliant psychological descriptions of madness stand in sharp contrast to Kraepelin's sterile attempts to pigeonhole the same behavior in medical terms. One of the very few physicians to contribute anything to the psychological view of man was William James and his contribution came only as he moved away from medicine into philosophy.

One other development at the end of the nineteenth century gave brief hope that the psychological stream might achieve maturity as an independent model for viewing man's behavior. In France, two new schools of psychiatry were emerging, a Salpetriere School under Charcot and a Nancy School under Bernheim. They both made hypnosis respectable once again, described and studied many conditions which were to be labelled as "neuroses," promoted the idea that many emotional disorders could be cured without exorcising devils or brain cells, and coined the term "psychotherapy" about 1890. Pierre Janet, another major French figure of this period, added the idea that neuroses were due to "subconscious fixed ideas" and advocated "automatic talking" (a precursor of free association) as a type of therapy. These men were within the medical tradition, but clearly stood in sharp contrast to the mainstream of medicine of their time. They strained the model, but they were not to prevail.

FREUD

The stage is set for the entrance of Sigmund Freud, the great codifier of the psychological model. And it is also set for the mistake—the categorization of the psychological under the medical model. Freud later realized his mistake, at least in part, but by then it was too late. The reasons for his mistake are easy to understand.

First, Freud was a doctor. Certainly he was a reluctant one—"neither at that time, nor indeed in my later life, did I feel any particular predilection for the career of a physician"[13]—but he was one nonetheless. He was a doctor in large part because he had little choice: "For a Viennese Jew the choice lay between industry or business, law and medicine."[14] He discarded the first two and only briefly considered the third. The faculties of law and medicine at the University of Vienna at that time both had a preponderance of Jews.[15] Ernst Jones, Freud's biographer, comments on his place in medicine: "He did not conceal in later years that he never felt at home in the medical profession, and that he did not seem to be a regular member of it."[16]

As a physician, Freud was strongly indoctrinated with the prevailing medical model for understanding human behavior. Two teachers who influenced him strongly were Brucke and

Meynert. For 6 years, Freud worked in Brucke's laboratory on the histology of the nervous system. His teacher had rather clear-cut views about human behavior:

> No other forces than the common physical-chemical are active within the organism. In those cases which cannot at the time be explained by these forces, one has either to find the specific way or form of their action by means of the physical-mathematical method or to assume new forces equal in dignity to the chemical-physical forces inherent in matter, reducible to the force of attraction and repulsion.[17]

Meynert, an eminent Viennese neurologist under whom Freud worked for 6 months, was convinced that depressions were caused by the overflow of blood in the brain.

Logically following his teacher, for whom he had reverent respect (Freud called Brucke "the greatest authority who affected me more than any other in my whole life"),[18] Freud proceeded to publish several papers on neurological subjects. He was becoming moderately successful as a neurologist and took pride in it: "I was able to localize the site of a lesion in the medulla oblongata so accurately that a pathological anatomist had not further information to add: I was the first person in Vienna to send a case for autopsy with a diagnosis of polyneuritis acuta."[19]

It is no wonder, then, that Freud's developing observations on irrational behavior were conceptualized in mechanistic terms compatible with medicine. His early writings read like a handbook of physics, with mental energy (especially "libido") having the properties of an electrical charge, being blocked by "resistances," and causing havoc if it were excessively dammed up. The unconscious was conceived of as a deep-seated organ operating with laws similar to those of physical energy. At some points, if you substitute the word "humor" for "libido," Freud begins to sound very much like the ancient Greeks. In an early work on neurosis, he says:

> All that I am asserting is that the symptoms of these patients are not mentally determined or removable by analysis, but that they must be regarded as direct toxic

consequences of disturbed sexual chemical processes, [specifically from] excessive masturbation and too numerous nocturnal emissions.[20]

So the first major reason for the mistake, the miscategorization under medicine of the psychological understanding of man, was that the master codifier of the psychological stream was a doctor strongly influenced by the medical beliefs of his age and by his teachers.

A related reason was the status of science during this period. Ernst Jones puts it succinctly:

> Moreover, in the nineteenth century, the belief in scientific knowledge as the prime solvent of the world's ills—a belief that Freud retained to the end—was beginning to displace the hopes that had previously been built on religion, political action, and philosophy in turn. This high esteem for science reached Vienna late from the West, particularly from Germany, and was at its height in the seventies, the time in question. Freud was certainly imbued with it, and so, despite his talents for exploring the unknown and introducing some sort of order into chaos, he must have felt that strictness and accuracy had an important place—visibly so in the "exact sciences."[21]

Freud was attracted to science because it was objective. He then spent much of his life trying to fit his theories of human behavior into a framework that would be acceptable to science. At times not only he but his followers have appeared obsessed with this goal. The failure of these efforts will become clear in later chapters. Their net effect at the time, however, was to push the psychological stream farther into the river of medicine, itself safely ensconced within science.

A third reason for the mistake was that much of Freud's early psychological theories concerned hysteria, a condition which mimics medical conditions. For instance, both an hysterical paralysis and a true paralysis are seen outwardly as an inability to walk. There the similarity ends: there is a vast difference between a person who cannot walk because of a conflict over his job and one who cannot walk because of brain damage.[22]

One can speculate on other reasons why Freud made the mistake of miscategorizing his psychological theories but they are less important. Though he did not feel at home in medicine, neither did he want to leave it. Doctors were held in very high esteem in Vienna at this period and it was not unusual to have streets named after them. Furthermore, his theories, with their emphasis on sex, were having a hard enough time making any inroads toward respectability in Victorian Vienna; at least medicine afforded them a modicum of protection. It is also significant that the men who had the greatest influence on his growth and thought were physicians—Brucke, Meynert, Breuer, and later Charcot and Janet.

Did Freud Have a Choice?

It is very easy to look back and say that Freud made a mistake by categorizing his psychological theories of human behavior under medicine. But in order to make a mistake, the element of choice must be present. If Freud had not tried to fit his theories into medicine, what else might he have done with them?

One possibility is that he might have started a new discipline altogether. He was not completely alone in his new explorations of human behavior: by 1880 there were at least seven books already written in Europe on the unconscious.[23] But to expect Freud to have stood by himself and to have fought for his theories as a new discipline is probably unrealistic. Freud was, after all, a Jew in an anti-Semitic, Catholic Vienna. Moreover, his theories centered on the importance of sex and this was also Victorian Vienna. Combined with the attraction he felt toward science and the influence of his doctor-teachers, Freud would have had to be extraordinarily perspicacious, brave, or masochistic to have tried to promote his theories as a separate discipline.

A logical alternative might have been philosophy. Freud was, by his own admission, strongly attracted to this field. In fact, during his first 2 years of medical school, he electively took five courses in philosophy, all under Brentano. In later years, he also acknowledged his debt to such philosophers as Fechner, Schopenhauer, and Nietzsche. Brentano was a well known professor of philosophy and psychology at the University of Vienna. If Freud had studied under someone else, he might have considered philosophy as an alternative home for his theories. As it turned out, however, Brentano strongly believed that both philosophy and psychology were part of science and that they would be fully accepted as sciences as soon as they could be proven to be based upon universal truths.[24] For Freud, then, it would have been nonsensical to have tried to fit his theories into a framework of philosophy if the framework itself was simply going to be subsumed within natural science. It made more sense, and was easier, to keep his theories within natural science from the beginning.

Religion was another possible framework but not a very attractive one for Freud. He was a nominal Jew, but not fanatical enough to try to interpret his theories as revealed truth. And certainly the Catholicism of Hapsburg Vienna was less than amenable toward his theories of human behavior which emphasized human sexuality. Moreover, religion was still linked with theories of possession, devils, and demons as explanations for illogical behavior and was therefore in complete disrepute among serious students of human behavior.

Finally, it might be thought that education would have offered a refuge for Freud's theories. He was, after all, talking of learning about yourself. And there was precedent, as Janet in Paris was evolving therapies of "emotional reeducation" and teaching "patients" how to live. Even in Vienna, Jacob Bernays, the uncle of Freud's future wife, had published a book in 1880 on Aristotle's concept of the theater as a cathartic learning experience.[25]

But Freud's personal education was such that by no stretch of the imagination could his theories fit into this framework. He was exposed exclusively to classical Aristotelian realism and Catholic Thomism. His final high school examination consisted of translations from German to Latin, Latin to German, Greek to German, mathematics, and an essay.[26] His major nonmedical teacher at the University, Brentano, was also an ex-Catholic who still followed the teaching methods of Aquinas. One of the philosophy courses which Freud took electively was Brentano's course on Aristotelian logic. For

Freud, then, education was simply a way of transmitting knowledge about things. It was not concerned with knowledge about people or knowledge about self. John Dewey, experimentalism, and progressive education were many years and many miles away.

In summary, it appears that Freud did have a choice of alternative frameworks within which to place his evolving theories of human behavior. None of them, however, offered very attractive options; and his mistake in choosing medicine is certainly an understandable one.

WHY HAS THE MISTAKE BEEN PERPETUATED?

The ring was closing. Before Freud, the irrational behavior of "madmen" had been quite firmly categorized as "disease." Now Freud claimed his new theories and methods were also part of medicine, so that hysterics too were categorized as "sick." It remained for his followers to apply his methods to a whole series of individuals who exhibited irrational behavior, each of whom then earned the label of "sick" if the methods showed any promise. The circle was closed by Harry Stack Sullivan in the twentieth century when he took Freud's methods and turned them back upon the original "sick" people, the "madmen" (mostly schizophrenics). His claim of success at "curing" these individuals effectively closed off discussion of whether psychological theories and methods were part of medicine; they had been "proven" to be so. Irrational behavior was "disease" and changing such behavior was "medicine."

It is useful to trace the developments which helped close the ring. Certainly there were counter-forces at all times trying to open up the categorization for questioning. For instance Groddeck, one of the early influential psychoanalysts, lectured his patients together on Saturday mornings in Zurich, suggesting that what he was doing was education. And Freud's followers numbered nonphysicians among the more important from the very beginning. Two of his original six "inner circle" (Hans Sachs and Otto Rank) were not doctors, nor were Theodore Reik, Anna Freud, Melanie Klein, Ernst Kris, Oscar Pfister, August Aichhorn, and many others.

But the forces tending to keep irrational behavior categorized within the medical stream were powerful. The most important of these are summarized:

1. Further medical discoveries

Ever since the end of the nineteenth century, there has been a series of medical discoveries which has suggested that human behavior would ultimately be explained simply as abnormal brain function. The effect of these discoveries has been to reaffirm the medical model and to tantalize the student of human behavior with promises of "ultimate truth" if only he would follow the medical path.

Syphilis was one of the greatest of these promises. In the late nineteenth century, it had been postulated that there was a disease of the brain which would explain the irrational behavior found among advanced cases of syphilis. In 1905 the spirochete was identified on the genital lesion and in 1913 it was shown to be present in the brain. The next 30 years saw the development of a series of cures for it, culminating in penicillin in the 1940s. The promise was seductive: "All ye students of irrational human behavior, wait long enough and all will be explained as this disease was!"

Many other medical observations and discoveries reinforced this message. The worldwide epidemic of influenza in 1917 resulted in many neurologically damaged people who showed irrational behavior and psychological changes as a result of this disease. Vitamin B deficiencies were shown to be associated with irrational behavior and "madness" in their late stages. Wilson's disease, phenylketonuria, and galactosemia pointed in the same direction. Studies of heredity apparently showed that causes of irrational behavior may be transmitted by the genes. And physical therapies such as electroshock, insulin shock, lobotomy, and most recently tranquilizing drugs have all suggested that irrational behavior is essentially a physical, anatomical, and medical entity.

2. Psychosomatic medicine

This is related to the first force, but it has been important in its own right in reinforcing the medical model of human behavior. The work of Walter Cannon showed how emotions produce physiological changes; for example, fear produces an outpouring of adrenalin from the adrenal glands. Other work has produced ulcers in monkeys by subjecting them to extreme stress and conflict. And in the 1930s, Flanders Dunbar's work, apparently relating specific medical conditions to certain personality types (e.g., an "ulcer personality"), became very popular. The establishment of the American Psychosomatic Association in 1939 put the official seal onto the inroads that psychiatry had been making into medicine. The reasoning went that if emotional stress can lead to physical disease and also to irrational behavior, then since the physical disease is part of medicine, the irrational behavior must be part of medicine too.

3. Kraepelinian classification

As noted above, once irrational behavior had been firmly classified, it made it easier to gain admission to medicine. This system of classification has remained in use (though useless) up to the present and has reinforced the medical model. There is a Rumplestiltskin mentality connected to its use—if you can name it, then you can understand it—but its effect is to make these "disease" categories of irrational behavior inviolate. Anyone who has doubted that irrational behavior is "disease" has only to look at his international classification of disease, find the correct code number for the behavior, and his doubts will be erased.

4. Mental hygiene and child guidance movements

These two movements arose in the first three decades of the twentieth century, the second being a logical outgrowth of the first. Both were an attempt to carry over the principles of public health to the field of psychiatry. Public health had shown great promise in decreasing such dread diseases as typhoid and tuberculosis. Why shouldn't it be equally effective in preventing the "diseases" of irrational behavior as well? The promise of these two movements reinforced the medical model, and it is only now that we are beginning to realize that they were but Pied Pipers. Irrational behavior cannot be "prevented" at all in the same sense that medical diseases can.

5. The Flexner Report

This may have been the single most powerful event which forced psychiatry to consolidate itself firmly within medicine. Abraham Flexner's 1910 report on medical education in the United States was a scathing exposure of the quacks and semi-trained doctors who were practicing medicine in the United States at that time. Its influence on American medicine was profound: the number of approved medical schools was reduced by half and professional standards were rigidified. This was badly needed at the time. The effect upon American psychiatry, however, was to produce a fanatical desire to get itself accepted by the medical establishment. Nobody but real doctors were allowed in the door lest they contaminate the "medical treatment" which was "psychotherapy." A. A. Brill, a leader of American psychiatry, even went to the New York State legislature and got a bill passed against lay analysts in 1926. And the American Medical Association issued a predictable warning about such nonmedical practitioners of a medical science. The desire for acceptance lasted through World War II, at which time the acceptance was mostly accomplished. It had taken medicine over 3,000 years to seize the province of irrational behavior from the fiefdoms of law, religion, and philosophy; once seized there was an obligation to protect it against nonmedical usurpers.[27]

6. The alternatives were not attractive

If irrational behavior is to be lodged elsewhere than in medicine, then the alternative must be attractive. We have seen that in Freud's time it was not. Over the next 50 years, it gradually became more so, especially the educational model which will be discussed later. Psychology proper, as an academic discipline, developed initially as but a handmaiden of psychiatry. Cattell's tests for memory and sensory stimuli were followed by Binet's tests for high mental functioning. Later Piaget and Rorschach added their dimensions, but it was not until almost the middle of the twentieth century that true clinical psychology developed and began to offer alternatives to the medical way of viewing human behavior. Unfortunately, just at this time, a major thrust developed within psychiatry to reincorporate clinical psychology in a handmaiden status, especially through the Veterans Administration hospital system. This has successfully inhibited the independent development of clinical psychology until the present.

FREUD QUESTIONS HIS MISTAKE

In the midst of these developments, there is much evidence that Freud himself had second thoughts about what he had done. At no point did he completely repudiate the medical model he had fought so hard to achieve stature in, but he did see it leading to some absurdities and he wanted to change it.

His doubts centered first on his role as a doctor. Ernst Jones described it as follows:

> I can recall as far back as 1910 his expressing the wish with a sigh that he could retire from medical practice and devote himself to the unraveling of cultural and historical problems—ultimately the great problem of how man came to be what he is.[28]

Historian H. Stuart Hughes also contends that Freud in later life had doubts about the rigid, scientific view of man that he had assumed earlier in his career. "The positivist vocabulary remained—but the positivist mentality had been largely sloughed off."[29] Freud was starting to see human behavior as not merely mechanistic and determined by pure laws of natural science. To the end, however, Freud clung to the belief that he was a scientist first and foremost, though clearly the evolution of his thought was making it increasingly difficult to hold to such a narrow base.

It was the controversy over lay analysts that most clearly brought out Freud's doubts about the medical model. As mentioned above, nonphysician (lay) analysts had been very important in the development of his theories from the beginning. These people were not doctors, yet they were practicing psychoanalysis and making major contributions to Freud's psychological theories. He realized that something was wrong with his medical model and fought bitterly for the acceptance of lay analysts. This fight "most keenly engaged Freud's interest, and indeed emotions during the last phase of his life."[30]

Freud himself is very clear on the subject:

> ...The internal development of psychoanalysis is everywhere proceeding contrary to my intentions away from lay analysis and becoming a pure medical specialty, and I regard this as fateful for the future of analysis.[31]

He never changed his mind on this. One year before his death he affirmed it: "The fact is, I have never repudiated these views and I insist on them even more intensely than before...."[32] Jones says that Freud believed it was "a matter of indifference whether intending candidates for psychoanalytic training held a medical qualification or not,"[33] and even urged such candidates not to bother with medical school:

> He envisaged a broader and better preliminary education for the novice in psychoanalysis. There should be a special college in which lectures would be given in the rudiments of anatomy, physiology and pathology, in biology, embryology and evolution, in mythology and the psychology of religion, and in the classics of literature.[34]

Freud lost this fight. He lost it partly because of the forces mentioned above, especially the influence of the Flexner Report on American psychiatry. At one point, American psychoanalysis even threatened to withdraw from the international association over the issue. And with the decimation of European psychoanalysis during World War II, the field was left to the Americans.

But Freud lost also because of the logical inconsistencies of his own thought. He wanted lay analysts yet could not give up the security of his medical model. He recognized his mistake and saw the problems arising from it; but in the end, he was too firmly wedded to his original paradigm to let go.

WHY IS PSYCHIATRY DYING NOW?

Given this long and multiplex history of how irrational behavior came to be categorized and perpetuated as mental "disease," why should things be changing now? Why is psychiatry—the medical model of human behavior—dying?

The main answer to this question comprises the substance of the next five chapters—the medical model of human behavior, when carried to its logical conclusions, is both nonsensical and nonfunctional. It doesn't answer the questions which are asked of it, it doesn't provide good service, and it leads to a stream of absurdities worthy of a Roman circus. Psychiatry is dying now because it has finally come to full bloom and, as such, is found not to be viable.

There are other less important reasons why psychiatry is dying now. One is that the sanctification of science and medicine has abated. We are no longer as certain that science will be able to solve man's problems; in some cases, it appears to have even made them worse. Medicine, sharing the mystical aura of science, is now viewed more as an effective set of therapies for the treatment of bodily diseases and less as a cure for all of man's problems.

Furthermore, two staunch defenders of the medical model—the Kraepelinian system of classification and psychosomatic medicine—are both in decline. Neither has realized the promise of its youth and both now find themselves quietly dreaming of their past days of glory. Another defender of the medical model—the Mental Hygiene movement—has evolved into the Community Mental Health movement. As will be shown, this movement is displaying too many Achilles' tendons to ever lead the medical troops.

Another reason why psychiatry is dying is that we are no longer under the cloud of the Flexner Report. Doctors generally are now ultrarespectable and psychiatrists stand near the top of the status ladder. No longer do psychiatrists have to use the servants' entrance; and as a result, we can afford to examine ourselves more critically. Related to this is a general movement within medicine to reexamine who does what to whom with what kind of training. This movement, stimulated by extreme manpower shortages and new career programs, has produced an atmosphere conducive to asking embarrassing questions about psychiatry and psychiatrists which in the past would have been considered heresy.

It should also be pointed out that by weight of sheer numbers psychiatrists have earned closer scrutiny. Thirty years ago, there were only 1,000 psychiatrists. Now there are over 25,000 of us and we are playing increasingly important roles in society. Whereas in the past we could be dismissed as a small group of eccentrics, we are now clearly visible. With this visibility has come the inevitable questions about what we do.

Finally, it should be repeated that the medical model cannot die until there are viable alternatives. As will be shown in Part II of this book, a modified educational model is one such possibility. Perhaps, then, psychiatry is presently dying because people for the first time are becoming aware of the possibilities of other models to explain irrational human behavior.

3

The Current Scene:
Systems of "Psychotherapy" as
Toothpaste

PERHAPS the most prominent feature of the current psychiatric scene is the existence of many varieties of "psychotherapy." Psychiatry is many other things as well—it is mental "disease," it is "hospitals," it is the legal exoneration of mental "patients" from responsibility, it is preventive mental "health." But above all, it is a mental "patient" contracting with a psychiatrist to get "cured" by "psychotherapy." This is how the majority of psychiatrists spend the majority of their time.

Of course many nonphysicians do "psychotherapy" too—psychologists, social workers, nurses, nonprofessionals. This in itself seems strange, since the very term "therapy" indicates that it is a medical procedure. Insofar as nonphysicians are carrying out medical procedures, they may be accused of practicing medicine without a license. Thus the fight of many psychiatrists to bar nonphysicians from practicing "psychotherapy" is solidly grounded in the medical model.

On the other hand, if "psychotherapy" is found not to be a medical procedure, then it need not be restricted to doctors. It should be renamed so that its semantic roots are planted in the correct soil. Then the qualifications for these who practice it could be drawn up in accordance with whatever kind of a procedure it is. This chapter will look at "psychotherapy" in an attempt to ascertain whether it is a medical procedure or not.

In scanning the scene, one notices immediately that there are multiple separate systems, each of which has a group of devotees claiming their system is the best one. On close examination, however, the systems of "psychotherapy" appear

rather like brands of toothpaste. Although each group of followers claims that their brand is best by virtue of some special color or flavor, in fact the base substance of all is found to
be the same. As I tried to show in *The Mind Game: Witchdoctors and Psychiatrists*,[1] "therapies" everywhere in the
world depend upon the same attributes for their effectiveness: a shared, world view between "therapist" and
"patient," the personality characteristics of the "therapist,"
the "patient's" expectations, and the techniques of "therapy."
Furthermore, what actually transpires in the "psychotherapeutic" situation is a process of education, not one of medicine. "Psychotherapy" is a medical procedure in name only;
in practice, it is an educational procedure. In light of this, it is
not surprising that all systems of "psychotherapy," like all
brands of toothpaste, get about the same results.

PSYCHOANALYTIC PSYCHOTHERAPIES

There are several different schools within this general
group, including orthodox Freudian, neo-Freudian, Jungian,
and Adlerian. Each of these schools in turn is further broken
down into subschools, e.g., the neo-Freudians are divided
into followers of Karen Horney, Erich Fromm, Harry Stack
Sullivan, and Frieda Fromm-Reichmann. Many of these
schools and subschools have their own training institutes. The
outcome is a panorama of parochialism and provincialism
not seen since medieval Europe.

In whatever ways these many psychoanalytic "therapies"
differ, they are all similar in trying to educate the "patient"
about his problems. As summarized in a recent textbook of
psychiatry:

> Analysis is essentially an educational process; it is a
> second education of adults and also of children and is
> supposed to correct the consequences of the traumas and
> faults of the primary education. It allows the individual
> to pay attention to the interconnections of his internal
> and private sensations and feelings. With the support of
> the analyst, the patient can update his earlier and private
> modes of experience and see himself and others with
> some new perspective.[2]

The content of the education varies slightly in the various schools and subschools, but most include information on what the person has stored in his unconscious ("where id was, there ego shall be"), the defense mechanisms and resistances the person uses, the importance of long-forgotten childhood experiences, and the way the person relates to certain adults (called the analysis of the transference). This education takes place slowly over many hours; for the more classical types, it may take 500 hours of private "psychotherapy" sessions before the education is judged to be complete. This being the case, it is not surprising that this kind of an education has strongly appealed to the intellectuals of the last four generations—it is the most complete education of the self that has been available.

In retrospect, finding that psychoanalytic "psychotherapies" are education rather than medicine should not be surprising. As seen in the previous chapter, Freud never intended that his "therapy" be administered by doctors alone. And many of the most significant contributions to these "therapies" have come from nondoctors.

Behavioral Therapies

A second major group of "psychotherapies" are those commonly referred to as behavioral "therapies." This group is also divided and subdivided into various factions which spend much time defending their particular boundaries. Some of the leaders of the behavioral "therapies" are physicians (e.g., Joseph Wolpe), although the majority are psychologists (e.g., Albert Bandura, B. F. Skinner, and Arnold Lazarus).

Of all forms of "psychotherapy," it is easiest to perceive the educational basis of this group. The theory upon which it rests is called learning theory and its literature is replete with concepts of learning and education. Proponents of behavioral "therapies" conceptualize not only the "therapeutic" process as a type of learning, but see the "disease" itself as a deficiency in learning. A phobia, for instance, is a product of maladaptive learning for a behavioral "therapist"; whereas for a psychoanalytically oriented "therapist," the phobia is an unresolved neurotic conflict.

The major types of behavior "therapy" are reward, punishment, desensitization, and negative practice. An example of a *reward type* is the practice in some state hospitals of giving the "patients" tokens for being able to care for themselves or to socialize with others. The tokens may then be cashed in for money or other rewards. Such a system is of course basic to classical techniques in education and a full token economy has even been tried in some classrooms.[3]

An example of a *punishment type* is the system called "aversion therapy," whereby a homosexual "patient" is shown two pictures, one of a nude man and one of a nude woman. Accompanying the first picture, he receives an electric shock. The outcome of such "therapy" is that a high percentage of homosexuals are said to be "cured" of their "disease."

The *desensitization type* of behavior "therapy" relies on the use of modeling behavior and overcoming fear in small doses. A child who has a phobia against dogs, for instance, is shown movies of people playing happily with dogs; then someone brings a dog into the room and plays with it; finally the child is asked to approach it slowly and pet it. The outcome is that the child loses his fear of dogs.

Finally, the *negative practice type* of behavior "therapy" involves overwhelming the "patient" with the object or situation which is most feared, and in this way reducing their fear. Thus a child with a phobia of water might be thrown into a swimming pool to overcome the fear.

Note that all of these procedures are labeled as "therapies," implying that they are medical, even though they are all based upon learning theory. This contradiction of terms has led to much confusion and argumentation among behavioral "therapists" themselves, some claiming that they are not related to medicine while others are holding onto the tenuous medical threads. What *is* clear conceptually is that these "therapies" involve a process of education and not a process of "curing."

ROGERIAN AND HUMANISTIC THERAPIES

The next broad group of "psychotherapies" to be considered are those of Carl Rogers and other humanistic psychologists such as Abraham Maslow and Rollo May. The Rogerian method of client-centered "therapy" will be discussed at length in a later chapter which will show that the focus on the personality attributes of the "therapist" have a counterpart in education. In fact, focusing on the personality attributes of the teacher (tutor) allows us to complete the educational model.

In addition to his client-centered "therapy," Rogers was also one of the architects of the humanistic psychology movement which has mushroomed into T-groups, sensitivity groups, and encounters all over America. Though this movement is not usually classified as "therapy" and therefore as part of the medical model, the line between it and group "therapy" is indistinct at best and some would say nonexistent. Both T-groups (the "T" stands for training) and "therapy" groups are composed of people who want to function more effectively, utilize a group leader with special training in group process, and operate with similar ground rules concerning self-disclosure and confidentiality. Both have also been shown to induce behavioral changes.[4] The major differences between the two kinds of groups are superficial—where they are held and how the people think of themselves. If the groups are held in a "hospital" or psychiatrist's office they are called "therapy" groups, whereas if they are held in a college dorm or someone's living room they become T-groups. Similarly, if the participants label themselves (or have been labeled) as "patients," they are "therapy" groups; otherwise they are T-groups. It would appear, then, that T-groups and "therapy" groups form a continuum and cannot be separated into neat medical and nonmedical compartments.[5]

It is also significant that the T-group movement is a direct offspring of education. The National Training Laboratory, parent organization and guiding force behind the T-group movement, has been affiliated with the National Education Association since its inception. Furthermore, the leaders of the T-group movement have themselves seen their product as an educational technique, not as a medical entity. For this reason, they have nurtured the growth of T-groups in such places as schools of education and schools of business, not in medical settings.

Another type of "psychotherapy" related to the humanistic psychology movement is what is called existential "psychotherapy." The juxtaposition of the two words themselves—existential and "psychotherapy"—provides an illustration of how far the medical model is being stretched in an effort to accommodate a nonmedical universe. Nevertheless, existential "psychotherapy" is included as a valid form of "therapy" in most recent textbooks of psychiatry.

According to Rollo May, "the central task and responsibility of the [existentialist] therapist is to seek to understand the patient as a being.... With it, the groundwork is laid for the therapist's being able to help the patient recognize and experience his own existence, and this is the central process of therapy."[6] This is a broad interpretation of the concept of "therapy" to say the very least. It makes much more sense to call it philosophy or self-education. One of the major reasons that it has achieved a medical standing sufficient to allow its admission into textbooks of psychiatry is that Karl Jaspers, one of the founders of modern existentialism, was a psychiatrist before he turned to philosophy. At any rate, existential "psychotherapy" is yet one more example of our attempts to fit the round pegs of self-education into the square holes of the medical model.

OTHER "PSYCHOTHERAPIES"

The various brands of "psychotherapy" discussed so far are all part of the mainstream of psychiatry and psychology. There are many other "therapies" which range from respectable to far-out, lunatic-fringe. Not all of them, of course, can be discussed here, but a sampling of them will suffice to ascertain whether they are medical or educational in nature.

One example is the system espoused by Albert Ellis, a "psychotherapy" which he calls "rational-emotive therapy." In this "therapy," the main emphasis is on thinking. The "patient" is told to let his intellect take precedence over his emotions and feelings. Ellis uses homework assignments for his "patients" in both individual and group "therapy." The role of the "therapist" in this system is to argue the "patient" out of his irrational beliefs, and to accomplish this often requires, according to Ellis, some lectures and a highly didactic approach by the "therapist."'

Another interesting form of "therapy" has emerged out of recent studies of what is called preventive psychiatry. This implies that it is possible to prevent people from becoming mentally "ill" if certain things are done. It has been found, for instance, that a person's ability to cope successfully with a crisis increases in direct proportion to his opportunity to anticipate and work through the crisis. Thus a person facing surgery is less likely to become mentally "ill" following surgery if he has the opportunity to discuss his fears and learn exactly what will happen during the procedure.

A kind of preventive "therapy" known as anticipatory guidance has been the basis on which Peace Corps volunteers have been counseled before going overseas. By having the volunteers anticipate and work through such feelings as loneliness, boredom, and frustration, which they will face, volunteers are theoretically better prepared to handle such conditions when they actually arise.[8] Anticipatory guidance has also been shown to be effective, in a controlled study, in helping foreign students adjust at an American university.[9] This "therapeutic" tool, of course, is nothing more or less than pure education.

A popular type of "therapy," promoted by Eric Berne and others, is the analysis of games.[10] In this "therapy," the "patient" is encouraged to become aware of the games he is playing in his social interactions. For instance, an alcoholic may have failed to achieve his life's goals. Instead of acknowledging the role that his drinking has played in the failure, he projects the blame onto his wife and plays "If it weren't for you!" "Psychotherapy" from Berne's vantage point becomes the analysis of social action with the goal of making the "patient" more aware of what he is doing.

A new type of "therapy" called money management "therapy" recently came on the scene.[11] It illustrates very clearly the absurd entities which the term "therapy" encompasses. The purpose of this "therapy" is to teach the mental "patient" how to manage his money. It can be done either individually or in group and is described as a "valuable complement to psychotherapy." If it teaches the "patient" how to pay his $40-an-hour bill, then I guess it certainly would be. Medicine has come a long way since Hippocrates.

Moving more toward the fringes, one can today find "therapies" that emphasize everything from screaming to tickling to punching. These are the new "body therapies."[12] Extraordinary as it sounds, people pay hundreds of dollars to be punched in the ribs or screamed at, all done in the name of "therapy." It really must be seen to be believed, with many of the group "therapy" sessions looking more like a karate parlor than anything else. These "therapies" rise and fall like pop songs and each month I await my issue of the popular psychology journals to see what "therapy"-of-the-month has arisen. The aim of them all is to teach the "patient" about his body.

Out on the far fringe, beyond the realm of respectability, one can find such forms of "psychotherapy" as sex. Doctor Martin Shepard, a well-trained New York psychiatrist and psychoanalyst, has published a book called *The Love Treatment* in which he details instances of sexual intercourse between "psychotherapists" and their "patients."[13] Dr. Shepard notes that "if the therapist's ultimate responsibility is to help his patient grow and learn, any and all means should be valid in reaching this goal." He then goes on to describe an assortment of heterosexual and homosexual relationships, including one in which a lawyer goes to a male "therapist" to get help with his marital problems and is seduced by him. But wait, that's just the beginning. At this point, the lawyer's wife joins the "therapy"; so the "therapist" recruits a male "co-therapist" who seduces the wife. And just like in the pornographic movies, they all have group sex, everyone feels better, and they live happily ever after. I believe this qualifies as "group therapy." The nicest touch of all, however, is that the government was paying the "therapists' " bills for the orgies.

Now one may suspect that Dr. Shepard is not serious, but that is wrong. The case is extolled as successful "therapy": it helped the lawyer "... to have friendlier relationships with men (unencumbered by fear of homosexuality) and allowed both [the lawyer and his wife] to deal with the question of fidelity in marriage." In what may be the most sophisticated rationalization of self-interest since man emerged from caves, sex is sanctioned as "therapy" and the medical model plummets to a new low.

Like all the other "therapies" discussed so far, the "therapist" conceptualizes what he is doing more in educational than in medical terms. Shepard says that "for me psychotherapy is in its ultimate sense an educative process." Not that responsible educators would claim his methods any more than responsible doctors would; nevertheless, like the other less "kooky" forms of "psychotherapy," it can be seen as a form of education.

THE COMMON BASE

Though this survey of types of "psychotherapy" is necessarily not complete, it does provide a sampling of representative brands. What, if anything, do they have in common? Is there any unifying feature among processes that stress insight into one's unconscious, learning therapy, sensitivity training, understanding one's own existence, the primacy of the intellect, anticipatory guidance, analysis of social games, the management of money, getting in touch with one's body, and even learning to fornicate?

One common element is that they are all labeled as "psychotherapy." Each has been stamped with a caduceus and put into the box marked "medicine," which amounts to an absurdity. These "therapies" have nothing in common with real therapies in medicine except the label. To categorize insight into one's unconscious with penicillin, renal dialysis, and an appendectomy is to approach asininity. You can stamp a caduceus onto Santa Claus's forehead, too, but that will not make him a doctor.

The more logical common base for all these activities would be the concept of learning—learning about oneself and others, about feelings, and about behavior. To learn is to acquire information, attitudes, and skills: information such as why a person reacts as he does toward certain people; attitudes such as the expectation of success rather than failure;

and skills such as handling interpersonal relationships.[14] As learning, these are all part of education, not medicine.

Many recent studies lead to the same conclusion. There are increasing attempts to extract the commonalities from different types of "psychotherapy." This is especially apparent in comparisons of psychoanalytic theory with learning theory, which almost invariably disclose that the two "therapies" are much more similar than dissimilar.[15] A recent symposium on the role of learning in psychotherapy came to the same conclusions, and there was a surprising amount of agreement on the function of learning as a common core of all "therapies."[16]

These attempts to extract the common elements from different forms of "psychotherapy" are all constrained from reaching full fruition by the medical model. It sits specter-like over the proceedings to remind the participants that they are still subjects of the medical domain. As long as this bird of Hippocrates retains its perch on the lintel, those who enter the room will have to continue to talk in the absurd language of "psychotherapy."

4

Mental "Disease" as Disease: Nymphomania Explained

IMAGINE that we have just placed a bet on a horse. The race begins and suddenly we notice that the jockey is seated backward on our horse. Now the horse can still run the race and he may even win. But until he does so, our confidence in our choice is seriously shaken by the jockey's odd way of riding. It is a distinctly bad beginning.

This is analogous to the position in which mental "disease" finds itself. The very term itself is nonsensical, a semantic mistake. The two words cannot go together except metaphorically; you can no more have a mental "disease" than you can have a purple idea or a wise space.

A mental "disease" is said to be a "disease" of the mind. Even the word "psychiatry" reflects this etymologically, being derived from the Greek *psyche* (mind) and *iatreia* (healing). But a "mind" is not a thing and so technically it cannot have a disease. "Mind" is shorthand for the activity and function of the brain. It is thinking, remembering, perceiving, feeling, wishing, imagining, reasoning, and all the other activities of which the brain is capable. Though we commonly use "mind" as a noun, we do so in a metaphorical sense and mean brain activity. Thus, "he has a good mind" means he can think or remember well; "pay him no mind" means not to pay attention to him; and "a piece of my mind" means what I am thinking. When "mind" is used as a verb, the idea of brain activity is clearer, as in "mind (pay attention to) your manners," "be mindful (aware) of..." and "I'm minding (caring for) my brother." The concept of "mind," then, can never be a place or a thing since it is activity and function.

The origin of the use of "mind" as a thing is clearly described by Ryle. He maintains that it arose as Descartes' myth, a product of the Cartesian dualism of mind and body. Ryle says "mind" is "the ghost in the machine" and that the concept "is entirely false, and false not in detail but in principle. It is not merely an assemblage of particular mistakes. It is one big mistake and a mistake of a special kind. It is, namely, a category mistake."[1] In this light, the mind-body dichotomy which has plagued medicine for generations is nonsense, as it opposes the body with the activity and function of the brain, part of the body. This is like creating a dichotomy between the whole of a car and the activity of its engine.

When we speak of the mind as if it were a place in the body, then we have used it as a metaphor. But when we drop the "as if," we start to believe it really *is* a place. Both Szasz[2] and Sarbin[3] have provided excellent analyses of the transition in the concept of "mind," first used as a metaphor but then reified into a thing. The mind became a mysterious place somewhere in the head, much as the "soul" became a mysterious place somewhere in the body.

A minor point, the reader may say, this mistaken reification of a metaphor. Surely a single solecism is not that important! But in fact, the mistake *is* important. We must be very clear on what we mean by a mental "disease" because our language shapes our thoughts. As Whorf and other linguists have clearly shown, language is the mold into which our thoughts are poured. If we forget that "mind" is only a metaphor, then it will shape our thoughts and determine our course of action.

Let me illustrate. In recent years, the medical metaphor has been used increasingly frequently to describe economic conditions. When unemployment and prices both rise, the economists often describe our economy as "sick." Facing inflationary dangers in 1969, President Nixon announced: "We are on the road to recovery from the disease of runaway prices."[4] Now everybody knows that runaway prices are not really a disease. But where this is forgotten, where the "as if" of the metaphor becomes lost, then something new occurs. We begin to think that runaway prices *are* disease. And if we are logical, we will assign a doctor to "cure" it. Absurd as it may sound, this is exactly what has happened in the field of human behavior.

MENTAL "DISEASE" AS BRAIN DISEASE

At this point, disciples of the medical model may answer: "What we really mean, of course, by mental 'disease' is brain disease. We mean that the structure and function of the brain are impaired." Brain disease, in this line of thought, is like kidney, liver, or thyroid disease. It is the impairment of structure or function of an organ. And by talking about brain disease, we are not in danger of creating another mysterious organ called the mind.

In fact, there are many known diseases of the brain, with changes in both structure and function. Tumors, multiple sclerosis, meningitis, and neurosyphilis are some examples. But these diseases are considered to be in the province of neurology rather than of psychiatry. And the demarcation between the two is sharp. Their union in the past was a marriage of convenience rather than desire; each has long since gone its separate way and developed its own friends. Their present relationship is confined to the ritual of joint specialty board examinations (soon to be discarded) and an occasional nod of recognition when they pass.

Furthermore, one of the hallmarks of psychiatry has been that each time causes were found for mental "diseases," the conditions were taken away from psychiatry and reassigned to other specialties. As the mental "diseases" were shown to be true diseases, mongolism and phenylketonuria were assigned to pediatrics; epilepsy and neurosyphilis became the concerns of neurology; and delirium due to infectious diseases was handled by internists.[5] In some cases, they have remained part of the psychiatric classificatory system; but in fact, the actual care of the disease has been transferred elsewhere. One is left with the impression that psychiatry is the repository for all suspected brain "diseases" for which there is no known cause.

And this is indeed the case. None of the conditions that we now call mental "diseases" have any known structural or functional changes in the brain which have been verified as causal. There is a presumption that structural and functional causes eventually will be identified. This is true not only for conditions with labels like "explosive personality" and "paranoid personality," but also for the behavior we categorize as "schizophrenia." And when specific structural or functional changes in the brain are identified—as they almost certainly will be for "schizophrenia" and other major "psychoses"— then these conditions will be given back to the neurologists to treat. Psychiatry will be left again holding the bag of brain "diseases" for which there is no known cause. This is, to say the least, a peculiar specialty of medicine.

It may be argued that even though we don't know the structural or functional defect for mental "diseases," we do know that there are chemical and neurological components and that it is therefore justified to call them true diseases. Certainly there are chemical and neurological components to an "obsessive-compulsive neurosis" or a "paranoid personality," but this does not make them into diseases. There are chemical and neurological components to *all* activities of the brain. Each thought, wish, memory, or impulse has a chemical or neurological component. This criterion by itself, therefore, is not sufficient to qualify a mental "disease" as a true disease.

The other argument commonly used to justify the concept of mental "diseases" as true diseases is the psychosomatic one. This focuses on the fact that there are psychological (mental) antecedents of many bodily diseases, e.g., ulcers, hives, and asthma. The reasoning is as follows:

1. There are psychological antecedents of bodily diseases.
2. There are psychological antecedents of human behavior.
3. Human behavior occasionally mimics bodily diseases.
4. Therefore, we are justified in labeling some human behaviors as mental "diseases" and putting them in the same class as bodily diseases.

To put this bluntly, the psychosomatic justification of the medical model is nonsensical. It is like saying parrots can move, cars can move, parrots sometimes mimic the sound of cars, therefore parrots should be treated like cars.

All we have said so far is that mental "disease" is semantically an intellectual abscess, a metaphor which has lost its "as if." The mind cannot *really* become diseased any more than the intellect can become abscessed. Furthermore, the idea that mental "diseases" are actually brain diseases creates a strange category of "diseases" which are, by definition, without known cause. Body and behavior become intertwined in this confusion until they are no longer distinguishable. It is necessary to return to first principles: a disease is something you *have,* behavior is something you *do.*

The semantic argument against mental "disease" as disease is a relatively minor one, however, compared to the others. The semantic inaccuracies could be excused if the concept was found to be functional. Let us see how functional the concept of mental "disease" is.

CLASSIFICATION OF MENTAL "DISEASE"

One of the attractive features of the medical model is the orderliness which accompanies it. In a culture like ours, where technology demands organization, labels and categories come to be sanctified. We divide, classify, catalogue, inventory, index, arrange, and file everything from groundhogs to toilet seat covers. Future archeologists uncovering the remnants of our civilization may decide that those few things which were not marked with an indelible pencil must have been valueless.

Medicine has accommodated itself to this need for order with aplomb. Diseases of the body are clearly and cleanly divided, either by the part of the body which is affected or by the cause of the disease. Thus, a general textbook of medicine is divided into chapters on diseases of the intestine, diseases of the circulatory system, and so on, as well as chapters on diseases caused by bacteria, diseases caused by allergies, diseases caused by chemical agents, and so forth. This compartmentalization is reflected in large hospitals by division into clinics along similar lines.

In its efforts to be included within the medical model, psychiatry has tried repeatedly to impose order onto its field and classify mental "diseases." Though attempts in this direction date back to Hippocrates,[6] it was Emil Kraepelin who created the definitive classificatory scheme early in this century. His work played an important role in solidifying psychiatry as a medical specialty. Kraepelin's original scheme has been extended, modified, and refined several times by the American Psychiatric Association, most recently in 1968.

The attempts to classify mental "diseases" along medical lines have been an embarrassment to psychiatry's friends and a delight to its enemies. Classification was not possible along lines of the part of the body affected, since presumably all mental "diseases" affect the brain in some way. Attempts to classify by the cause of the disease ran afoul of the fact that the cause was not known.

So psychiatry has shuffled, cogitated, debated, and emerged with a classification system that is a semantic jungle. Mental "diseases" are officially classified using eleven different criteria. When a mental "disease" is to be classified, one must consider the following:

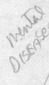

mental DISEASES

1. Causative agent (when known)—e.g., chronic brain syndrome due to syphilis
2. Intelligence—e.g., mental retardation
3. Certain personality traits—e.g., explosive personality
4. Age—e.g., adjustment reaction of adolescence
5. Sexual behavior—e.g., homosexuality
6. Habits—e.g., bed-wetting
7. Parts of the body presumably affected by the "disease" of the brain—e.g., psychophysiologic cardiovascular disorder
8. Emotions—e.g., depressive neurosis
9. Relative sobriety—e.g., acute alcohol intoxication
10. The proximity of the person to his domicile—e.g., runaway reaction
11. Whether the person is breaking the law—e.g., group delinquent behavior

This is an incredible mishmash of labels when analyzed. Systems of classification are supposed to help sort, order, and divide items. But the sorting criteria used by psychiatry are such that everyone fits into some categories and most people fit into several of them simultaneously. Rather than sorting diseases, the classificatory system merely provides an arbitrary assignment of labels for behavior. It is the facade of classification without the substance. In this system, it would even be possible to have an adolescent, mentally retarded boy with congenital syphilis who has problems with bed-wetting and homosexuality. At a point where he drinks some beer and runs away from home with other boys, all eleven labels above might apply to him simultaneously.

The absurdity of the classification of mental "disease" has not been lost upon psychiatrists themselves. Karl Menninger has dismissed the most recent classificatory efforts as "sheer verbal Mickey Mouse."[7] Another psychiatrist's reaction to the section on children's mental "disease" is that it "...can only be termed unscientific and bordering on the ridiculous."[8] The points of weakness in the classification are unlimited; one may ask, for instance, if the normal effects of aging on the brain are to be labeled as a disease ("senile dementia"), then why is there no similar disease category for the state of the brain of infants? In trying to make logical sense of the classification of mental "diseases," I have a recurring fantasy of a group of dwarfs sitting in the forest trying to decide whether apples should be classified with tomatoes because they are red, with balls because they are round, with chestnuts because they grow on trees, or with watermelon because they are fruit.

Since numerous studies have shown the low reliability and limited predictive value of systems for classifying mental "diseases,"[9] in practice they are usually ignored. Except on legal documents such as insurance claims, in court, and for the purpose of statistics, most psychiatrists do not use formal diagnostic labels in their day-to-day practice.

Two explanations for this programmed confusion are possible. The first is that it is only because psychiatry is "young" that our classificatory system is so inadequate. Proponents of this view argue that the system will improve as more causes of mental "diseases" are discovered.

The other possibility is that something is inherently wrong with the task—that maybe mental "diseases" are not diseases at all in the medical sense. If so, then all attempts to classify mental "diseases" are futile and other ways must be found to classify human behavior. The value of classification is not the issue: we cannot transmit knowledge without categories. What *is* being questioned is the functionality of the medical model as a basis for classification.

THE CAUSE OF NYMPHOMANIA

A hallmark of physical diseases is that they usually have clear-cut causes. A bacteria which causes pneumonia, a fall which causes a broken leg, a deposit of fat which causes a heart attack—all are, at least, partial explanations for the disease process which follows. And, as mentioned previously, knowledge of these causes provides the basis for classifying physical diseases.

In an attempt to achieve parity with their older and more distinguished brothers, mental "diseases" have striven to attain this same kind of causal respectability. Freud focused on early infantile experience, especially sexual, as the important causal agents of later "disease." Subsequently, other psychiatrists have emphasized biological, familial, or social causes of mental "diseases." In all cases, however, the medical model demands a cause (or causes) for the "disease." As summarized by one recently trained psychiatrist: "The medical model does apply to the treatment of mental illness, which is the product of a complex of infantile wishes just as real and potentially treacherous as the primary tubercle complex."[10]

It was only this medical model of mental "disease" that enabled me to understand the recent trial of a nymphomaniac in San Francisco.[11] A twenty-nine-year-old businesswoman had sued the Municipal Railway of San Francisco for injuries caused to her in a cable car accident. It seems that the accident had caused her to contract her mental "disease" of nymphomania and she sought $500,000 in damages.

The woman had been raised as a devout Lutheran by strict Midwestern parents. Details of her "pre-disease" personality centered on her days as a choir girl and her two "affairs of the heart" as a university coed. Then in 1964, she was a passenger on a cable car which rolled backward and crashed. She was thrown against a pole, suffering bruises and "psychic injuries." The accident was said to have "shattered her security." The pole which she was thrown against was equated with her stern Lutheran father and this somehow caused severe "psychic trauma."

The result of this accident was said to be nymphomania. At the time of her trial, she admitted to having had over 100 lovers since the accident and, at one point, having engaged in sexual intercourse fifty times in 5 days. She was distressed by her own promiscuity and described herself in her diary as "a human garbage can." Her attorney described her as "a fallen sparrow." During her 20-day trial, four psychiatrists and seven other "medical experts" testified on her behalf. In addition, her attorney subpoenaed six of her many lovers to verify the sequence of events, as well as the cable car gripman. The defense countered with a single psychiatrist. A jury of four men and eight women deliberated 8 hours and awarded her $50,000. Her attorney was said to be distinctly disappointed with the outcome, as the psychiatrists had testified that treatment of this "disease" might cost up to $30,000 a year and take as long as 5 years.

This trial seems at first glance incredible, but it *is* logically consistent with the medical model of mental "disease." If indeed nymphomania is a disease, then it must have a cause. And given the present state of our knowledge, the sequence of events as outlined cannot be proven false. A private investigator working for the plaintiff summarized it as follows: "The accident *was* responsible for her condition. Suppose she had broken her leg on the cable car. Would there be any question of damages?" And in his closing remarks, her attorney said: "This jury can proclaim that people who have injuries of the mind have injuries far more serious than injuries of the body." This extension of the medical doctrine of causality into the realm of litigation and compensation opens up a cornucopia of possibilities—public transportation would become uninsurable and some homosexual men could sue their overprotecting mothers.

There is precedent for invoking such causal connections in suits which involve mental "disease." Another example is the case of the twenty-three-year-old airplane mechanic who shot and killed his girl friend in a premeditated murder to which he confessed.[12] In reply to the question whether he fired with intent to kill (he shot her nine times), he replied: "I fired to blow her fucking head off. How many times do you want me to tell you?"

Despite this straightforward admission, he was examined by a total of nine psychiatrists and three psychologists to determine his sanity. They concluded that he had a mental "disease" consisting of a desire to be punished. That "disease" had been caused by guilt over his father's death, who was killed in a fall while chasing his son, then age nine, to make him wear a hat to school. The jury was not impressed and the defendant was found guilty of murder and sentenced to death.

Both of these cases show how traumatic events can be utilized as causes of mental "disease." If in fact, there *is* any validity to this medical model, it should be verifiable. One attempt to do this was an experiment where ten senior psychiatrists, ten psychiatric residents, and ten laymen were asked to examine the significant life experiences ("dynamic formulations") of thirty-four psychiatric case histories. They were then asked to place the case into one of seven possible diagnostic categories. In other words, by knowing the important causal agents in the history, could they predict the type of mental "disease" that the "patient" would have?

The results were uniformly negative. All three groups did the task with only slightly greater than chance ability and there were no statistically significant differences among them. The author of the study concluded:

> This study clearly challenges the idea that it is meaningful to discuss specific life experiences as predisposing to a given illness. Dynamic psychiatry has failed to predictively discriminate between individuals with similar past experiences who later become neurotic, psychotic, or remain asymptomatic. It is suggested that the medical formula of assigning etiological significance to specific constellations of past events has limited applicability with respect to comprehending mental illness.[13]

Like the classification of mental "disease," it is possible to say that we just don't know enough about the causation of mental "diseases" to make predictive statements. In this view, it is only a matter of time before we will. The alternative view is that there is something grossly wrong with the model itself and we will never be able to make such predictive statements. In this view, the causation of nymphomania by a cable car accident will look just as absurd 100 years from now as it looks now.

This is not to deny for a moment that there are psychological antecedents to human behavior. There certainly are—traumatic experiences, deprived childhood, and so on may contribute to disturbed human behavior in later life. This is qualitatively different, however, from saying that the traumatic experiences are "causes" of a disease as if the experiences were bacteria. As is apparent in the cases cited above, the imposition of the medical model has important legal consequences.

DIAGNOSIS AND CATCH-22

Medical conditions are, for the most part, "clean." You either have them or you don't. A broken arm usually shows up on X-ray. Pneumonia is diagnosed when the clinician hears certain sounds in the lung through his stethoscope. A person is diagnosed as a diabetic when the level of his blood sugar exceeds a certain threshold. Medical texts contain abundant tables of "normal values" and the working assumption is that when a person deviates from these figures then he is sick. There are always some cases where equivocation about the diagnosis is needed; but even there, the equivocation is more about *what* the person is sick with, not whether or not he is sick.

In its attempts to follow the medical model, psychiatry has longed for clean mental "diseases." It has experimented with various diagnostic criteria to determine "disease," but all attempts to date have failed miserably. Probably the most common method is to try to differentiate "neurotics" and "psychotics" from normals and these two terms are usually used as if they are two different "disease" categories.

Criticism of them by psychiatrists has been abundant. It is said that there is no general agreement on what criteria must be present to make such diagnoses. Different psychiatrists usually set their own criteria and may include such data as the suspected cause of the "disease," the overall clinical picture, the quantitative and qualitative differences in symptoms, the course of the "disease," the proportion of the person's personality which is involved, the place of treatment, and predictions about the future course of the "disease." As two psychiatrists summarize it: "It has become increasingly evident in recent years that the traditional classification of mental illness as psychoses and neuroses is no longer useful, even administratively, because of the wide variation and growing confusion in the definition and use of the terms."[14]

This was seen very clearly when Rosenhan, a psychologist at Stanford, had perfectly sane people admitted to 12 different mental hospitals simply by telling the admitting psychiatrist that they were hearing voices.[15] The voices were saying things like "empty, hollow, and thud" (the experimenter, with a fine sense of humor, decided that he would create "an existential psychosis"). Otherwise, these normal people, mostly graduate students, gave completely truthful histories to the psychiatrists. They were all diagnosed as "schizophrenic," except one who was diagnosed as "manic-depressive." Once admitted, they acted perfectly normally; yet were held for 7 to 52 days (the average was 19) and were given over 2,100 pills total. The true patients on the wards often recognized them as pseudopatients but the staff never did. Once labeled, the staff's perception of them was apparently so profoundly colored that normal behavior was seen as part of their psychosis.

In an even more damning postscript to the experiment, Rosenhan told one hospital what he had done. He then told them that he would try to gain admission for another pseudopatient there within the next 3 months. Ever watchful for the pseudopatient who was never sent, the staff labeled 41 of the next 193 admissions as suspected pseudopatients; over half of these were so labeled by a psychiatrist. The experimenter concluded: "Any diagnostic process that lends itself so readily to massive errors of this sort cannot be a very reliable one."

Another serious challenge to the neurosis-psychosis dichotomy as diagnostic criteria for mental "illness" came from a research study of prestige suggestion.[16] In this study, a psychiatrist taped an interview with a professional actor. The actor was told to play the role of a healthy, normal young mathematician "who was enjoying life, who had read a book on psychotherapy, became intellectually curious, and wanted to see if it would help him enjoy life even more fully." According to the researchers, the actor "quickly established a warm interpersonal relationship with the interviewer, cordially verbalizing his inner experience in a coherent and organized fashion, without evasion, defense, withdrawal, or guilt."

The tape of this interview was then played to five groups of people:

   a. 156 undergraduates enrolled in a course in clinical psychology
   b. 40 law students
   c. 45 graduate students in clinical psychology
   d. 25 practicing clinical psychologists
   e. 24 clinical psychiatrists

Each of the groups was told that the man was a young mathematician who had come into the clinic out of intellectual curiosity, as outlined above. They were then told that "although he looked neurotic, he actually was quite psychotic" and that a prestigious person in their field had verified this. Following this, the tape was played and the listeners were asked to diagnose the "patient." The following are the results:

| | PERCENT OF ANSWERS | | |
GROUPS	Psychosis	Neurosis or character disorder	Normal or mild problems
Undergraduates	30	54	16
Law students	14	76	10
Psychology graduate students	11	77	12
Clinical psychologists	28	60	12
Clinical psychiatrists	60	40	0

It is clear from the results, as the authors state, "that prestige suggestion may bias diagnosis" and that "psychiatric diagnosis is a process of labeling social behavior." In control groups where the suggestion was not given, the majority diagnosed the "patient" as normal and none thought he was psychotic. Most surprising, perhaps, is the finding that "prestige suggestion had most effect upon psychiatrists, biasing them in the direction of psychosis, least effect upon graduate students; clinical psychologists fell between these extremes and both of these groups made significantly more diagnoses of neurosis and health than did psychiatrists."

This experiment is only one in a long series of experiments which have shown the low reliability of psychiatric diagnosis. In one instance, thirty-five separate patients were interviewed by three psychiatrists jointly. The psychiatrists agreed upon the major diagnostic category 46 percent of the time and upon the specific diagnosis only 20 percent of the time.[17] In other instances, only two psychiatrists were used, it was not possible to get agreement on the specific diagnosis more than 55 percent of the time.[18] A variation on this theme was Pasamanick's experiment showing that two psychiatrists on the same ward seeing the same group of patients over a 2-year period differed in their diagnosis of "schizophrenia"; one psychiatrist diagnosed it in 22 percent of the patients and the other in 67 percent. Pasamanick concluded:

> These findings provide concrete statistical affirmation for the view that despite protestations that their point of reference is always the individual patient, clinicians in fact may be so committed to a particular psychiatric school of thought, that the patients' diagnosis and treatment is largely predetermined. Clinicians, as indicated by these data, may be selectively perceiving and emphasizing only those characteristics and attributes of their patients which are relevant to their own preconceived system of thought. As a consequence, they may be overlooking other patient characteristics which would be considered crucial by colleagues who are otherwise committed. This makes it possible for one psychiatrist to diagnose nearly all of his patients as schizophrenic while an equally competent clinician diagnoses a comparable group of patients as psychoneurotic.[19]

The consequences of these wide discrepancies among clinicians can be seen in the percentage of inductees rejected on psychiatric grounds during World War II. Although the test scores on psychological tests were approximately the same from induction center to induction center, the percentage of recruits who were declared unfit for service varied from 0.5 percent to 50.6 percent among the different centers.[20] In light of such findings, it may be seriously questioned whether the process of diagnosing mental "diseases" deserves to be called diagnosis at all in the medical sense of the word.

Another criterion which has been tried for the diagnosis of mental "disease" is that of contact with reality. If the person is not in contact with reality, then he is defined as mentally "ill." Conversely, if he *is* in contact with reality, then he is not mentally "ill," at least not as severely.

The pristine logic of this criterion for the diagnosis of mental "illness" was immortalized by Joseph Heller in *Catch-22*. In that book, he has Yossarian follow it to its conclusion in his attempt to get himself diagnosed as "crazy" and therefore relieved of further flight duty:

> Yossarian looked at him soberly and tried another approach. "Is Orr crazy?"
>
> "He surely is," Doc Daneeka said.
>
> "Can you ground him?"
>
> "I sure can. But first he has to ask me to. That's part of the rule."
>
> "Then why doesn't he ask you to?"
>
> "Because he's crazy," Doc Daneeka said. "He has to be crazy to keep flying combat missions after all the close calls he's had. Sure I can ground Orr. But first he has to ask me to."
>
> "That's all he has to do to be grounded?"
>
> "That's all. Let him ask me."
>
> "And then you can ground him?" Yossarian asked.
>
> "No. Then I can't ground him."
>
> "You mean there's a catch?"
>
> "Sure there's a catch," Doc Daneeka replied. "Catch-22. Anyone who wants to get out of combat duty isn't really crazy."
>
> There was only one catch and that was Catch-22, which specified that a concern for one's own safety in the

face of dangers that were real and immediate was the process of a rational mind. Orr was crazy and could be grounded. All he had to do was ask; and as soon as he did, he would no longer be crazy and would have to fly more missions. Orr would be crazy to fly more missions and sane if he didn't but if he was sane he had to fly them. If he flew them he was crazy and didn't have to; but if he didn't want to he was sane and had to. Yossarian was moved very deeply by the absolute simplicity of this clause of Catch-22 and let out a respectful whistle.

"That's some catch, that Catch-22," he observed.

"It's the best there is," Doc Daneeka agreed.[21]

Psychiatrists too have been impressed by the apparent simplicity of this criterion and invoke it readily to justify a diagnosis. As in *Catch-22*, however, they frequently encounter inconsistencies and absurdities when they try to use it.

For example, there is a large social factor which enters into consideration in using this diagnostic criterion. Certain people under certain circumstances are allowed to be out of contact with reality without being diagnosed as mentally "ill." For others, the diagnosis seems to follow automatically if they betray thoughts that are not readily accepted by other members of the society.

An illustration of how social circumstances affect this criterion for mental "illness" is offered by the case of oleomargarine heir, Michael Brody. Early in 1970, he received national publicity by declaring that he had $25 million that he was going to give away. In one of his ventures, he went to the White House:

Brody arrived at the White House in a taxi and, instead of paying the driver, promised to send him enough money to live on for the rest of his life.

Then Brody turned to reporters and announced: "The war in Vietnam is over and the North Vietnamese troops have gone home." He said he learned of the war's end by "superior intelligence" and has 500 jet planes stationed at various points around the globe "ready to fly the boys home by Saturday."[22]

Now it may be questioned whether Brody was in contact with reality as he stood next to the White House. However, when listening to a person who supposedly has $25 million, it is unusual to doubt his veracity. Probably anyone else who made such a statement in those circumstances would find themselves immediately hospitalized for observation to detect mental "illness." Brody was merely called eccentric.

The social factor present in diagnosing mental "illness" is in contrast to physical illness. Had Brody coughed up blood, he would be suspected of having tuberculosis no matter how much money he had. And a broken arm is a broken arm in all social ranks. The fact that diagnosis of mental "disease" often depends upon social considerations casts further doubt on the validity of the criteria used for diagnosis.

Who Is Normal?

Normality is another aspect of the medical model which has caused problems for psychiatry. The medical profession has always had quite explicit ideas about which persons are considered normal. If a person does not have a disease, then he is normal. An arm looks normal on X-ray if there is no fracture, lungs sound normal if there are no sounds in them except for breath sounds, and a person's blood is considered normal if the cell count is within certain limits. Thus normality for medicine is the absence of disease; this definition has been widely accepted since the time of Hippocrates.

Psychiatry, in its attempts to become a subdivision of medicine, has been troubled by this definition of normality. In trying to define normality as the absence of disease, it has found itself in an awkward position. The reason for this is that there is no accepted definition of mental "disease." As stated by Jahoda's monograph for the Joint Commission of Mental Illness and Mental Health, "...no satisfactory concept of mental disease exists as yet and...little would be gained by defining one vague concept in terms of the absence of another which is not much more precise."[23] In short, we cannot define normality as the absence of mental "disease" because we do not know what mental "disease" is. This argument in itself suggests how unsatisfactorily the medical model fits the field of human behavior.

Jahoda, in fact, dismisses the medical approach to normality in just five pages. She says that psychiatry must develop and utilize other approaches and goes on to describe six "promising" criteria. These concepts, it should be noted, are drawn from the work of nonphysicians like Maslow, Erikson, Allport, Rogers, and Fromm. The rejection of the medical model is so complete in this monograph that Dr. Walter Barton, the Medical Director of the American Psychiatric Association and one of the members of Dr. Jahoda's advisory panel, felt it necessary to append a dissenting chapter to the report titled "View-point of a Clinician." In it he reaffirms the classical medical position that mental health and normality are "the absence of disease."[24]

Psychiatrists have made other attempts to define normality by evading and avoiding the medical model. Psychoanalysts, for instance, conceptualize normality as a utopian state which we can never reach—a goal to be striven for.[25] This approach is well represented in the works of Freud himself who was fond of pointing out the slips of the tongue in everyday life. Thus everybody was said to have some "psychopathology." Another approach is one of functionalism, where normal is defined in the social context of the person's ability to function.[26] This and other concepts of normality will be returned to later; the point to note here is that either explicitly or implicitly they all reject the medical model of normality as inappropriate.

In instances where a medical approach to normality and mental "disease" have been utilized, the results have often been amusing, sometimes absurd. The classic instances of this have been the field studies which have tried to measure the incidence (or prevalence) of mental "illness" in a given population. For instance, the Midtown Manhattan Study in New York City found that of the people in the lowest socioeconomic stratum less than 5 percent were mentally "well." Almost half the people they studied had "mild or moderate symptom formation" and the other half were even worse. If normality is the absence of disease, then less than 5 percent of

this population is normal.[27] Similarly, Leighton's studies in
Nigeria and Nova Scotia found that 42 percent and 47 percent (respectively) of the people studied were "sick" with psychiatric "symptoms."[28] Lest the reader think that all this
mental "illness" is confined to New York City, Nigeria, and
Nova Scotia, a study of children in affluent Westchester
County, N. Y., found that two-thirds of the children suffered
from "emotional impairment" and that only one-third were
"emotionally healthy."[29] Normality, in these studies, takes on
the character of an exclusive club to which only a select few
may belong. And mental "disease" becomes an angry plague,
stalking the land and infesting whole populations.

The other instance where the medical approach to normality is used consciously and purposefully is in the lobbying for
mental "health" funds in Congress. This began with the post
World War II investment of the federal government in mental "health" and mental "disease." It was argued that 10 percent of all World War II draftees had been rejected on the
grounds of mental "disease" and another 10 percent of those
drafted had had to be hospitalized for similar reasons. The
numbers game has since become perfected by both professional and lay mental "health" groups so that all requests for
money are liberally sprinkled with quantitative rhetoric of
"patients," costs of "treatments," and the gross discrepancies
between supply and demand.

In fact, if we were to follow logically the medical approach,
almost everybody would be mentally "ill." The present official classification of psychiatric "diseases" is already so broad
that there is a real question whether anybody can claim to not
fit into at least one category. To do so, one would have to be
free of everything from anxiety, depression, suspiciousness,
and hostility, to ulcers, asthma, and hives, to tics and disorders of sleep, to acute alcohol intoxication. In short, all you
have to do to qualify as "normal" under the present system is
to be a bowl of jello.

But things may get worse. Serious and respected thinkers in
psychiatry have suggested that the concept of mental "disease" be broadened. One psychiatrist would even include

grief as a disease, reasoning that the loss of a loved one is a causative factor of disease "...of such general importance as to be put in the same class as other major noxa, e.g., physical agents, microorganisms, etc."[30] Reflecting on the logic of this, I am reminded of the series of items in which the test subject is asked to find the item which doesn't fit, e.g., red, blue, cat, yellow, orange. In this case, the list might be cancer, diabetes, grief, pneumonia, typhoid fever.

One of the results, then, of the medical approach to mental "disease" is that everybody ends up qualifying as mentally "ill." The spectre of mental "disease" haunts us and becomes "the nation's number one public health problem." It is even more prevalent than hemorrhoids.

5

Mental "Disease" as Curable: "Doctors," "Hospitals," and the Mad Hatter

"DOCTORS" who are not doctors and "hospitals" which are not hospitals comprise the world of psychiatry. It is a setting worthy to host the Mad Hatter's tea party. Instead of "Why is a raven like a writing desk?" we might ask "How is a psychiatrist like a doctor?" or "How is a mental hospital like a real hospital?"

Doctors and hospitals are integral parts of the medical model. Doctors are the designated agents of cure and their role presupposes some training. Even when someone other than a doctor (such as a nurse or medical corpsman) treats a patient, it is still expected that a doctor is ultimately in charge. Similarly, hospitals are places for people who are seriously ill. These institutions, known for over 1,000 years, serve to provide diagnostic and therapeutic services for the patients.

Both "doctors" and "hospitals" are used by psychiatry, but in name only. They are vastly different from their counterparts in medicine and these differences shed further light on the nature of psychiatry. If basic concepts like "doctors" and "hospitals" are found not to apply to psychiatry, then what parts of the medical model *do* apply?

"DOCTORS" WHO ARE NOT DOCTORS

The first and most striking thing about the practitioners of psychiatry is that many of them are not medical doctors at all! As mentioned previously, this has been true from the very beginning of psychiatry. Otto Rank and Hans Sachs in Freud's "inner circle" were not physicians, nor were such later figures as Theodore Reik, August Aichhorn, Ernst Kris, Oscar Pfister, Melanie Klein, and Anna Freud. This impressive group of nondoctors has more recently been augmented by others such as Anatol Rappaport, Rollo May, Bruno Bettleheim, Erich Fromm, and Erik Erikson. Nor does this list include all the psychologists whose work has profoundly influenced psychiatry—men like Carl Rogers and Albert Bandura. The fact that so many leaders of psychiatry are nondoctors is revealing of the true nature of psychiatry.

Exactly how important nondoctors are in leadership roles was quantified by Rogow in his recent survey of American psychiatrists. In response to the question, "Who are the most outstanding living psychiatrists and psychoanalysts?", the first and third choice for both psychiatrists and psychoanalysts were nondoctors—Anna Freud and Erik Erikson. Only the second choice of each group was a doctor (Karl Menninger and Heinz Hartmann respectively).

Another indication that psychiatrists themselves are willing to ignore a lack of medical training among their leaders was illustrated by the reports of the Joint Commission on Mental Illness and Health. This prestigious body was set up by the official psychiatric and mental "health" organizations to assess the state of psychiatry. They published a series of ten monographs; of the twenty-three combined authors of these monographs, only three—3—were medically trained psychiatrists. Such a degree of nonmedical participation is totally inconceivable in surgery, obstetrics, or any other of the true medical specialties.

Psychiatrists, although medical doctors, also differ remarkably little from other psychotherapists—psychoanalysts (some of whom are not doctors), psychologists, and psychiatric social workers. All four are alike in their family and social background; e.g., in all four groups, approximately half are Jewish and two-thirds are brought up in a large city. The similarities of medical psychiatrists with nonmedical psychotherapists is so striking that it has been proposed to group them all together as "the fifth profession."[2]

Furthermore, the general public is not concerned in most cases whether the person caring for them is a psychologist (without a medical degree) or a psychiatrist (with a medical degree). It is the eternal fate of all psychiatrists to be so confused and they can count on having to explain the difference at least once at each cocktail party they attend. The percentage of the general public who can make this distinction is very small; the percentage who care is even smaller. This in itself suggests something about the irrelevancy of a medical education for a psychiatrist.

The next curious thing to note about psychiatrists as "doctors" is in the realm of what they do. They never touch their "patients." This is indeed an extraordinary way to practice medicine. If anything is really wrong with the "patient" physically, then the psychiatrist will call in an internist, surgeon, or whatever; but he will not examine the "patient" himself. The exceptions to this are rare and are frowned upon by the profession.[3] I can clearly remember one of my supervisors confiding to me during my training that he sometimes patted his "patients" on the back on their way out of the office. Horrors! If discovered, he may be branded as an infidel.

Another indication of the official confusion (some would say "flexibility") on psychiatrists as "doctors" is reflected by psychoanalysis. In 1937, the American Psychoanalytic Association clearly stated that psychoanalysis was a medical procedure and therefore that psychoanalysts must be doctors. Eight years later, they redefined it as education so that it would qualify for inclusion under the G. I. Bill for returned veterans of the war. Presently, psychoanalysis is a medical procedure for a housewife who may take it as a tax deduction for medical expenses and an educational process for an internist who may deduct it as a business expense (for improving existing skills). A "medical" procedure which may be viewed so many different ways is certainly a remarkable procedure! As Thomas Szasz summarizes it, "...the tax status of analysis belongs with Alice in the realm of Wonderland."[4]

"Doctors" Who Avoid Really "Sick Patients"

Another peculiarity of psychiatrists as "doctors" is that they avoid the really "sick patients." Instead, they spend the vast majority of their time with those "patients" who are least "sick." This is certainly a curious way to practice medicine.

CAMROSE LUTHERAN COLLEGE LIBRARY

In medicine in the United States, it is generally acknowledged that the sickest patients are in hospitals. This is presumably also true for psychiatry. But that is not where psychiatrists are. Over the past 20 years, the total number of psychiatrists has quadrupled in this country. Today, however, there are *fewer,* in total number, psychiatrists working in public mental "hospitals" than there were 20 years ago.[5] For instance, Searcy State Hospital in Alabama had one licensed physician for every 372 "patients" in the early 1900s. In 1968, it had one licensed physician for 2,200 "patients." This is not unusual in the United States, but it is indeed a strange phenomenon. It is as if the number of surgeons had quadrupled over the past 20 years but there were now fewer surgeons to treat hospitalized cases of fractures, ruptured appendices, and inflamed gall bladders.

This manpower deficiency at the points of greatest need is also seen in other segments of psychiatry. For instance, of the 2,000 psychiatric outpatient clinics in the United States, *two-thirds* of them do not have a single full-time psychiatrist on their staff.[6] And in our 160 penal institutions with a total of 146,662 inmates—a group frequently characterized as seriously mentally "sick"—there are a grand total of less than 100 psychiatrists.[7]

The fact that psychiatrists are not spending much time with the "sickest patients" can also be seen in the results of a recent survey.[8] When the percentage of total psychiatric manhours was tabulated for various practice locations, the results were as follows:

State mental hospitals	14%
Community mental health centers	7%
Institutes or schools for the mentally retarded and/or the emotionally disturbed	1%
Correctional institutions and prisons	1%
Drug addiction and rehabilitation centers	0.4%
Alcoholism centers	0.2%
Nursing homes	0.1%

According to the rhetoric of the mental "health" movement, it is in these locations that the "sickest patients" are to be found. But it is clear that this is not where many psychiatrists are to be found. By contrast, 41 percent of psychiatric man-hours was spent in private offices and another 13 percent in private and general hospitals. The remainder was spent in teaching, research, and administration.

The way that psychiatrists spend their time, and the discrepancy between supply and demand, is best illustrated by a recent study done by Ryan in Boston.[9] This city provided an excellent setting for such a study because it has one of the highest concentrations of psychiatrists—250 of them—anywhere in the world. If a mentally "ill" person cannot get adequate care in this city, then it is doubtful he can anywhere. Ryan found that of every 1,000 people who had contact with social agencies in Boston, 150 were identified as "emotionally disturbed." Of this 150, only 10 ever received help in a mental "health" setting and only one of them by a psychiatrist.

When Ryan surveyed the psychiatrists to see what they were doing, he found that only 20 percent of their "patients" could be classified as "seriously ill." The psychiatrists were seeing between twenty and thirty new patients per year. These patients were typically young, college-educated people who were only mildly "ill" compared to their neglected counterparts in the "hospitals." In fact, about one-quarter of all private psychiatric patients in Boston are young women in their twenties and early thirties who live within an area of less than 100 blocks. This certainly must rank as the strangest and most exclusive "medical" practice since all physicians were confined to the courts of kings in the Middle Ages.

When we turn our sights on psychoanalysis, the situation becomes even more absurd. Most of these practitioners have 3 to 5 years of training in psychoanalysis beyond that of a regular medical psychiatrist. They should, in theory, be our most skillful "doctors" for treating mental "disease."

So how do they spend their time? According to a survey conducted by psychoanalysts themselves, less than 9 percent of their "patients" are seriously ill enough to be called "schizophrenics." Their patients are 98.8 percent white and 78 percent college-educated or higher.[10] Another study of 144 "patients" under the care of 30 psychoanalysts revealed that one-third of the "patients" were derived from the mental "health" profession itself and *none* of them was diagnosed as "psychotic." Furthermore, the nonmedical nature of "treatment" is suggested by the fact that only 2 of the 144 "patients" received medication during the year of study.[11] A full-time psychoanalyst, using classical Freudian techniques, can only see *eighty* patients in his *total 30-year practice*. It is doubtful if even a king in the Middle Ages would tolerate *this* as a "medical" practice from his most highly trained "doctors."

It can also be shown that psychiatrists are distributed in a geographical pattern which corresponds with their "treatment" pattern. They are clustered in areas with large numbers of wealthy people who can pay for the "treatment" and they are virtually absent in lower socioeconomic areas. For instance, Westport, Connecticut, is a wealthy suburb of New York City; it has 30 psychiatrists for its population of 30,000. By contrast, the Chicago suburban areas of Gary-Hammond-East Chicago have a blue collar population of 600,000 and only 7 psychiatrists. One has a psychiatrist-to-population ratio of 1 to 1,000; the other has a ratio of 1 to 100,000. Another example of this is New York City's affluent upper East Side where two adjacent buildings contain the offices of sixty-five psychiatrists; this is more than can be found in any one of sixteen states. Psychiatry is the only "medical specialty" with such gross discrepancies in the distribution of its practitioners; the reason is that it is not really medicine.

"DOCTORS" WHO DO NOT "CURE"

Diseases of the body are for the most part curable. Some, like pneumonia, can be completely cured with antibiotics. Others, like diabetes, can be controlled with insulin and thus cured in the sense that symptoms are alleviated. Even for those bodily diseases which cannot be cured—for instance, lung cancer—there is general agreement that a cure would include either control or eradication of the tumor. The concept of cure in medicine, then, is reasonably clear and generally agreed upon.

Psychiatry, by contrast, has been unable to arrive at any such general consensus on what "cure" means. This is not surprising in view of the difficulties psychiatry has defining "disease." But attempts to define "cure" for these "diseases" quickly become submerged in a river of ridiculosity.

Some psychiatrists avoid the dilemma altogether by refusing to talk about "cures." In their general textbook of psychiatry, for instance, Redlich and Freedman say: "As a rule, however, the use of the term cure in psychiatry is not appropriate."[12] This is, of course, illogical and inconsistent with the medical model; if you talk about "disease," then by definition you must include the concept of "cure" as well.

The problems of psychiatry begin when attempts are made to define a "cure." Most definitions revolve around the goals of "therapy" which are being striven for; when these goals are reached, then the person is said to be "cured." Now for the person with pneumonia, the goals of therapy are clear—eradication of the disease organisms, removal of the symptoms, and usually the return of the individual to full function. For a person with a mental "disease," the possible goals of "therapy" include a much broader spectrum. Some of the possible goals are the following:

1. Symptom removal, e.g., reduction in anxiety
2. Attitude change, e.g., "right-mindedness" stressed in Eastern therapies
3. Behavior change, e.g., stopping of compulsive handwashing
4. Insight, e.g., understanding why you are depressed
5. Improved interpersonal relationships, e.g., getting along with your neighbors
6. Improved personal efficiency, e.g., greater ability to accept responsibility
7. Improved social efficiency, e.g., greater ability to do socially useful work
8. Prevention and education, e.g., increasing the ability to adapt and cope in future situations

These goals of "therapy" for the "cure" of mental "disease" differ significantly from the goals of therapy for the cure of bodily diseases in that they are much more closely related to the values of that culture. For instance, some values held in high esteem in the dominant culture in the United States are work, achievement, independence, responsibility, and rational thinking. The predominant goals of "therapy" for mental "patients" are, therefore, insight, improved personal efficiency, and improved social efficiency.[13]

Other cultures, by contrast, hold other values in high esteem and thus may have different goals of "therapy" for their mental "patients." The Navajos, for example, place harmony within the community as the greatest value; the most important goal of "therapy," therefore, is improved interpersonal relationships. This is accomplished most often by a long "curing" ceremony which involves the whole community. It has been described as follows:

> A significant implication of this [Navajo] view is that the patient does not need to reflect on his behavior or examine his motives, conscience, or reactions in order to be helped. There is no exhaustive analysis of intrapersonal dynamics; he need only place himself within the curing system, which, once set in motion, proceeds almost automatically.... In one sense, all Navajo curing is psychotherapy. Looked at another way, however, none of it is psychotherapy as we know it. In the sense of verbal interaction between patient and therapist, with the goal of changing behavior through increased insight and self-awareness, psychotherapy hardly exists at all.[14]

In Japanese culture, one dominant set of values is based upon Oriental philosophy and patterned after Zen Buddhism. The idea striven for is a calm but happy acceptance of reality. For a Japanese mental "patient," therefore, the goal of "therapy" which is most important is "right-mindedness," a change in attitude:

> In such terms, the goal and problem of psychotherapy for the Japanese is how to live in the midst of this sad transitoriness of all things—one does not struggle against this, but becomes one with it. There is no need to look backward as in Western psychotherapy to seek for past causes which no one can prove to have really taken place.[15]

In Japan, this is often accomplished by a particular combination of techniques called Morita therapy, which includes rest, solitude, the daily study of the "patient's" diary, and occupational therapy.

The point is that "cures" really do not exist for psychiatrists in the same sense as for other doctors. For psychiatrists, a "cure" is a relative, strongly culture-bound concept. A New York psychoanalyst faced with a depressed Navajo or Japanese individual is virtually useless. A New York internist faced with a pneumonia-stricken Navajo or Japanese individual can cure him quite effectively with penicillin.

There is additional evidence to challenge the concept of "cures" in psychiatry. It appears that not only is "cure" a culture-bound concept, but it is class-bound as well. Different observers have shown that the goals of the mental "hygiene" and mental "health" movements are not absolute, biological goals. Rather they are cultural values that coincide with those of the group who are dominating the movement. Kingsley Davis demonstrated this over 30 years ago when he showed that the ideas of the mental "hygiene" movement coincided remarkably closely with the ideals of proper Protestant Bostonians. Coincidentally, the movement at that time was almost entirely dominated by proper Protestant Bostonians.[16] More recently, others have shown that the values espoused by the current mental "health" movement are predominantly middle-class values and that "...the mental health movement is unwittingly propagating a middle-class ethic under the guise of science."[17] This indictment holds for the entire concept of "cure" of so-called mental "diseases."

DOCTORS WHO DO NOT NEED TO BE TRAINED

A final and perhaps most curious thing about psychiatrists as doctors is that they apparently do not need to be trained in medicine. Individuals who have not been so trained appear to get about the same results as the psychiatrists do in their practice of "psychotherapy."

This fact has been revealed in gradual stages over the past 25 years and the full realization still has not taken place. It began during World War II when clinical psychologists (not medically trained) were pressed into action in Veterans Administration hospitals. They performed more than adequately the tasks which had been the exclusive domain of psychiatrists and they have continued to do so ever since. Then, in the 1950s, social workers began going into the practice of "psychotherapy" and the results paralleled those for psychologists.

The 1960s brought the paraprofessionals and new careerists to the mental "health" scene and they repeated the success of the psychologists and social workers. Studies have been done with college students, housewives, medical corpsmen, hospital aides, and just indigenous neighborhood residents, showing that they obtained about the same results as the professionals using "psychotherapy" with "patients." One such study, for example, compared college students with psychiatrists and psychiatric social workers doing group therapy with hospitalized psychiatric "patients." The college students got the best results.[18]

If psychiatrists do not need to be trained as doctors to do their job, then what kind of training do they need? It is clear that some training is desirable.[19] The optimal kind appears to be that which increases insight into other people's problems and the ability to help other people change their behavior. In short, training in the behavioral sciences—not in medicine—is what is needed. Probably equally as important, however, are the personality characteristics of the person who is the "therapist," the sharing of a world-view between the "therapist" and the "patient," and the expectations of the "patient."[20] Psychiatrists, then, who turn out to be good "psychotherapists" do so in spite of, not because of, their medical training.

Many psychiatrists will concede the above points readily but will still insist that medical training is very important, or even essential, for being a good "psychotherapist." Three major rationales (or rationalizations) for this are usually proffered. The first of these is that "psychotherapy" is based on science and, because of this, its practitioners should be trained in the scientific method in general and medical science in particular. In response to this argument, one must first ask whether "psychotherapy" is really scientific. "Scientific" in our culture means "good"; it is a value judgment as much as a method. We try to persuade others that whatever we do is scientific, from making a better beer to being a "psychotherapist." In the land where laws of motion are kings and chi square is the court of last resort, we dutifully appeal to science as the ultimate justification for psychiatrists being doctors. In fact, as I have tried to show elsewhere, the techniques used by psychiatrists are no more scientific than those used by their counterparts—medicine men, shamans, and witchdoctors—around the world.[21] Furthermore, the scientific method is certainly not confined to medicine; chemists, physicists, psychologists, and other nonmedical persons use it as well. Therefore, there is no substance to this argument, either on the ground that "psychotherapy" is scientific or on the ground that only doctors use the scientific method.

An interesting experiment which further adumbrates this argument (if more is needed) was an attempt using a programmed teaching method to teach college freshmen enough psychiatry to pass the psychiatric part of the National Board Examination.[22] This examination is taken by most graduating medical students and is supposed to test the emerging doctor's knowledge of psychiatry. The nineteen college freshmen who tried the experiment studied an average of 12.3 hours; their average score on the examination was over 61 percent. One individual studied only 3 hours and got a 62 percent. If this is any reflection on the amount of scientific substance in the learning of psychiatry, then the amount of it must be meager indeed. It is inconceivable that results such as these could occur with any other medical specialty on the National Board Examination.

Another rationale given for the medical training of "psychotherapists" is that since medical diseases often contribute to mental "diseases," then the person treating the latter had better be a doctor so that he can recognize the medical components. This argument has some truth to it and its proponents are quick to invoke studies which show that between one and five percent of mental "hospital" admissions really have a medical disease masquerading as a mental "disease." This is true and certainly some screening procedure is needed to differentiate such individuals. However, since the psychiatrists themselves are mostly not working in the mental "hospitals" anyway, it would seem that their practice belies their argument. It is also quite possible to develop an adequate system which would not require medically trained psychiatrists to screen individuals presenting behavioral problems; the signs and symptoms of possible organic brain disease can be taught to a nondoctor in one or two weeks for screening purposes.

It should also be noted that medical disorders contribute to many things besides mental "diseases," yet the same conclusion is not drawn. For instance, disease and injuries are of crucial importance to a baseball or football team; yet we do not require the coach of these teams to be a doctor. All he has to do is to be able to recognize when it is necessary to call in a doctor. Thus the fact that medical disorders contribute to other activities does not in itself justify the conclusion that the activity should be in the charge of a doctor.

A third reason given for the medical training of "psychotherapists" is that only doctors understand how to truly take responsibility for another human being. Such responsibility, it is claimed, is part of medical training and, as such, justifies psychiatrists being trained as doctors. This is an important issue and it is often used as the ultimate argument to justify the medical model.[25] There is some truth to it but there is also some falsehood. There are many psychiatrists who do not take responsibility for their "patients" and there are many psychologists who do. The taking of responsibility may not be a function of the training at all, but may be related to factors of preselection, i.e., more responsible individuals may be attracted to medicine. Why cannot people be selected for this trait and then be encouraged to develop it further? The successful use of lay people in mental "health" settings (e.g., the thousands of housewives presently staffing suicide prevention centers) have shown that responsibility is a commodity on which medicine does not control the market.

"Hospitals" Which Are Like Prisons

Turning from doctors to hospitals, one is confronted with another panoply of parodies on the real thing. Hospitals are old and respected institutions for the care of people seriously

ill. These institutions provide intensive diagnostic and therapeutic services for the patients, enhancing the chances for
cure. They are also, of course, a convenience for doctors and
other agents of cure insofar as they concentrate patients in
one place. Hospitals have proven to be very useful institutions for medicine and have been partly responsible for its
remarkable progress in the past 200 years.

Logically following the medical model, psychiatry also established places wherein serious mental "diseases" should be
"cured" and called these places mental "hospitals." The common rationale for their use is that they provide a setting for
the intensive "diagnosis" and "cure" of mental "disease," that
they provide a place for mentally "ill patients" who are
unable to maintain themselves outside of the "hospital," that
they protect a "dangerous patient" from himself (i.e., suicide),
and that they protect society from "dangerous patients." Let
us see how they function.

The first thing to be noted is how different mental "hospitals" are in overall structure from regular hospitals. Sociologist Irving Goffman did a lucid analysis of this in *Asylums:
Essays on the Social Situation of Mental Patients and Other
Inmates.*[24] He compares mental "hospitals" with prisons, concentration camps, army barracks, boarding schools, monas-
teries, and sanitariums for tuberculosis and leprosy. All, he
contends, are "total institutions" where "a large number of
like-situated individuals, cut off from the wider society for an
appreciable period of time, together lead an enclosed, formally administered round of life." Goffman shows very
clearly that the most important determinants of the behavior
of a "hospitalized" mental "patient" are due to the fact of
being "hospitalized," not to being mentally "ill." Thus, a
mental "hospital" is much more like a prison than like a regular hospital. This is recognized in some states, such as Ohio,
where both kinds of institutions are under a single Department of Mental Hygiene and Corrections.

Mental "hospitals" are also like prisons in that the inmates
have contravened socially acceptable behavior and have been
found guilty of doing so. There is little doubt whether they

are guilty or not—their very presence in the prison or "hospital" is accepted as implicit proof. As summarized by Maisel in a very perceptive article,

> Once a person has been admitted to a hospital for observation, it is very difficult for him to convince the staff that he is not "sick." There are several reasons for this "presumption of illness." First, both the apprehending agents and the hospital staff generally agree that certain types of socially disturbing behavior express a pathological state of mind, a "mental illness." Second, "habitual" behaviors are defined by law as grounds for confinement in a mental hospital; the charge of mental illness need not be proven, or even considered. Third, the process by which a person becomes a mental patient helps to create new evidence for mental illness: confusion and shock leading to withdrawal, resistance, or apathy. Finally the staff is expected to discover "symptoms" of mental illness, however subtly expressed, and to note them in the hospital record.[25]

Maisel concludes that mental "hospitals" are "convenient centers for housing, either temporarily or permanently, persons who have proved troublesome to society, who have habits that are either self-destructive or socially bothersome and who have provoked others into doing something about them."[26]

In terms of length of inmate stay, mental "hospitals" are not only like prisons—they are much worse! It should be noted that there are over twice as many inmates in mental "hospitals" in this country as there are inmates in prisons.[27] And they stay in the mental "hospitals" much, much longer. In New York State mental "hospitals," three-quarters of the inmates have been there longer than 2 years. In all federal prisons, only one-quarter of the inmates have been there longer than 2 years.[28] A recent survey of St. Elizabeth's "Hospital," the federal mental institution in Washington, D.C., revealed that *37 percent* of the inmates had been there *longer than 20 years.*[29] Less than two-tenths of one percent of inmates in federal prisons have been there that long. Even in a prison like Leavenworth where the incorrigible are sent, the average inmate has been there only 2½ years.[30]

The upshot of this is that convicted criminals are quickly learning what might be called the McMurphy Rule (from Ken Kesey's novel about a man who gets himself transferred from a prison to a mental "hospital" for a softer life and ends up getting a frontal lobotomy instead).[31] This rule states that if you have to be an inmate somewhere, always opt for a prison over a mental "hospital."

"Hospitals" with Strange "Treatments"

The institutions which are called mental "hospitals" have spawned, over the years, a predictable and consistent series of horror stories about what goes on in them. They are, in fact, a sure-fire story for any newspaperman who is looking for a quick headline; and this has been consistently true for almost 100 years. One of the more recent such exposés was that of Partlow School for the Mentally Retarded in Alabama which was alleged to be "not even providing custody because custody implies safekeeping. Partlow was providing storage."[32] Specifically, it was said that some of the "patients" were not known by name by anyone on the staff and that a drug order which was supposed to have been given for 7 days was still being given 3 years later.

One may protest that such outrages of human care have nothing to do with medicine or the medical model. But they may. By calling the inmates of these institutions mental "patients," we insist, by definition, that doctors, nurses, and other medical personnel must be found to care for them. This is of course unnecessary—most mental "patients" need some kind of human care but not necessarily medical care. And, in fact, the best (and often the only) care given in these "hospitals" usually come from some of the lower-level, underpaid "aides." Doctors are almost never seen. As calculated by one observer, a mental "patient" in an average mental "hospital" in 1961 experienced person-to-person contact with a physician for only 15 minutes each month.[33]

One of the most frightening consequences of such medical staffing was the case of Ricardo Munoz-Velez, a Cuban refugee who worked as a doctor at Elgin State "Hospital" in Illinois. As explained by the *Chicago Tribune:*

> When he was chief of pathology at Elgin State Hospital, Ricardo Munoz-Valez demonstrated total medical incompetence in working with corpses. So, mental health officials demoted him by transferring him to the hospital wards where he treated live patients.[34]

And treat patients he did, with "...inappropriate drugs and dosages, homespun cures of boiled potatoes and bananas for choking patients, and archaic treatments."[35] Certainly such individuals are not typical, but the fact that they can occur at all is a poignant commentary on our institutions called mental "hospitals." It should also be noted that it is the necessity to staff these "hospitals" with "doctors"—a direct consequence of the medical model—which makes it possible for a Cuban with questionable medical credentials to be put in charge of "patients."[36]

Another highly questionable "treatment" which is inflicted on mental "patients" is psychosurgery (e.g., lobotomy). The only justification for it is, of course, the medical model. When an appendix is diseased, it is cut out; therefore, when a portion of the brain is "diseased," it may also be cut out. Far from being a thing of the past, psychosurgery has made a comeback and is currently being done on 400 to 600 "patients" a year in the United States.[37] Along the same lines, electrode implants in the brain have been used to treat Parkinson's disease (a tremor of the hands). Why not also use electrode implants to treat mental "diseases"? The man who has pioneered experimental work in this field sees no reason not to use them on people who are too aggressive, criminals, and juvenile delinquents.[38] And, of course, he is right. Insofar as we are willing to call such examples of human behavior mental "diseases," we are obligated to try medical treatments which have proven of value in other medical diseases. Don't be squeamish now—once we get your electrode in place, you'll feel much better about the whole thing.

But even accounts of psychosurgery pale beside descriptions of what a psychiatrist can do to a mental "hospital" armed only with his medical model and an electroconvulsive therapy machine. It is horrifying because it is so inexorably logical once one accepts the basic tenets of the medical model. One such description is that of an American psychiatrist who took over a South Vietnamese mental "hospital" to modernize it with recent advances from American psychiatry. This account is from the pages of the respectable *American Journal of Psychiatry.*[39] It makes Kesey's novel read like the Bobbsey Twins.

First, the psychiatrist decided that all the "patients" must do some work. The incentive which he used to get them to work was to offer electroconvulsive therapy (ECT) as the alternative. He refers to this modern American psychiatric technique as "operant conditioning therapy." On the men's ward, he obtained good results, i.e., most of the men decided to work. But when he tried his "therapy" on the women's ward, he had much less success. Out of a ward of 130 women "patients," he forced only 15 of them to go to work after twenty ECT treatments.

Not to be defeated by the failure of his first "therapy," he initiated the next—work or starve! Unless the women went to work, he refused to give them any food. The psychiatrist proudly reported that all the women were finally working after only 3 days of starvation.

Now one may call this incredible "hospital" an aberration and say that the psychiatrist is misguided to put it very mildly. But note the logic of the justification which he uses:

> The argument that subjecting these patients to electro-convulsive treatments or withholding food might be considered cruel was countered by the comparison to a child with pneumonia receiving antibiotic injections. The injections hurt and even involve some slight risk to the patient, but the damage without their use is potentially much greater. Inflicting a little discomfort to provide motivation to move patients out of their zombi-like states of inactivity, apathy, and withdrawal was, in our opinion, well justified.

It is the medical model and he is perfectly right. If these

"patients" are "sick" partly because they are apathetic and inactive, then in "curing" them it is important to reactivate them. The psychiatrist himself reports the results of his "therapy" as very successful: "Results demonstrated the remarkable effectiveness of this technique for motivating patients to resume productive activity."

It should be added that the "productive activity" which this good doctor arranged for his discharged "patients" was to be hired by the Green Berets to fight against the Vietcong. And for those who might be upset by the doctor's "treatment" method he adds: "The use of effective reinforcements should not be neglected due to a misguided idea of what constitutes kindness."

HOSPITALS IN WHICH SOME PEOPLE WANT TO STAY

The next important thing to note is the composition of "patients" in mental "hospitals." In contrast to regular hospitals where patients with diabetes, pneumonia, and broken legs fill the beds, the people admitted to mental "hospitals" fall into three groups:[40]

a. 25 percent are senile, older people who have lost the ability to function because of the natural changes of age
b. 50 percent are alcoholics, "neurotics," "character disorders," and lonely people
c. 25 percent are labeled as "psychotics" (most of whom are called "schizophrenics"); these people are said to not be in touch with reality

These "patients" differ from those in regular hospitals in many important aspects. One of the most important is that many of them *want* to be there. Moreover, some even want to stay indefinitely. I was first struck by this when, as a resident, I was assigned to a ward in a Veterans Administration hospital. In all my experience in regular hospitals, I had not had any difficulty discharging patients. Almost all of them, when told they could go home, would eagerly put on their clothes and depart smiling. Now I was suddenly in a peculiar kind of "hospital" where "patients" pleaded to stay and where the direct threat I had at my disposal was to discharge someone.

Little John illustrated this Alice-in-Wonderland state of affairs clearly. He had been a "patient" on the ward for 5 years, having first been admitted for stabbing himself superficially in the chest. He went to his job in the "hospital" every day, did his share of work on the ward, was given weekend and holiday passes, and had banked $10,000 in government pensions during his stay. When I suggested to him that he might be discharged, he immediately told me how depressed he felt and that he might try to commit suicide again. A previous attempt to discharge him had even been blocked by the director of the "hospital" because of the suicide threats. I counted it a major accomplishment of my 6 months at this "hospital" that I successfully moved Little John to another ward.

This is anything but an isolated case. Mental "hospitals" contain large numbers of Little Johns, a fact tacitly ignored by everyone concerned since it is in both the "patient's" and the "doctor's" best interests to ignore it. The only analysis of this phenomenon of which I am aware is an excellent book called *Methods of Madness: The Mental Hospital as a Last Resort.*[41] In it, the authors use nine tests to show that the "patients" in a state mental "hospital" act just like the rest of us. Almost all the subjects they tested had been labeled as "psychotics":

> We may find it peculiar that some persons would se-
> lect such a milieu in the first place, but what they do
> once inside is no more ineffectual or irrational than the
> activities of any other community of persons. It is ex-
> traordinary how predictable (and sensible!) the conduct
> of patients becomes once one assumes that, for the most
> part, they want to remain in the hospital and that they
> know what they are about![42]

Another aspect of this is what is called the "blacklist." This is a list of former "patients" which a mental "hospital" will not readmit because of their destructive, threatening, or predictably inebriated behavior. Most mental "hospitals" keep such a list of potential "patients" and woe be unto the unwary doctor who mistakenly admits one. The existence of such a "blacklist" at all is quite extraordinary *if* these places are really hospitals. Presumably, the behavior which gets the person into trouble in the "hospital" is the same behavior which necessitates his "hospitalization" in the first place. It would be like making a blacklist of ulcer patients who bleed too much or have too much pain.

"HOSPITALS" IN WHICH PEOPLE GET "SICKER"

Another fallacy about mental "hospitals" which is frequently used to justify them is that they protect society from large numbers of "dangerous mental patients." In fact, the number of individuals in these "hospitals" who can be considered as dangerous is infinitesimal. Most "patients" who have committed crimes are not put in regular mental "hospitals" but rather are sent to special institutions for the "criminally insane." These are, to all intents and purposes, just prisons with a hospital label.

Evidence points strongly toward the fact that mental "patients" are *not* dangerous, contrary to our stereotype. In "patients" followed up after their discharge, studies have almost unanimously shown a lower arrest rate than that of the general population. For instance, one follow-up of 5,883 discharged mental "patients" showed an arrest rate of 6.9 per 1,000 arrests compared with 99.7 for the general population.[43] A similar study of 10,247 patients revealed an arrest rate of 122 compared with 491 for the general population. The only study to the contrary is one from Maryland which showed discharged mental "patients" to have a higher arrest rate for robbery and about the same arrest rate as the general population for the crimes of assault, rape, manslaughter, and murder.[44] One researcher summarizes the evidence as follows: "It might be said that these patients who have left mental hospitals are not as dangerous to the community as those who have never been judged mentally ill."[45]

Even in the case of the criminally "insane" (the very name strikes terror in our hearts and makes us recheck the bolt on the front door), there is evidence that we have magnified their dangerousness all out of proportion. The U. S. Supreme Court provided a natural way to find out when, in 1966, they handed down an unexpected decision which resulted in the abrupt transfer of 967 "patients" from New York State "hospitals" for the criminally "insane" to regular mental "hospitals." These "patients" were commonly said to be the most dangerous mental "patients" in the state; and to find out, they were followed-up for 5 years. During that time, only 26 of them had to be returned to a "hospital" for the criminally "insane." Half of the group went on to be discharged from the mental "hospital"; and of these, 83 percent had no further arrests.[46]

It would appear from such studies that mental "hospitals" are being used for preventive detention of many people whom we fantasize are dangerous. The actual figures belie our fantasies—they are not really any more dangerous than most of us are. In fact, if we rationally wanted to lock up potentially dangerous people, we would not release any convicted felons from prison; for it is known that they have a re-arrest rate of up to 80 percent. But we do not and should not; felons serve their prescribed sentences and then are released. We abide by the tenet that it is not justified to lock up people for something they *might* do, for this is an infringement on our freedom.

But not so with mental "patients." They are kept for indeterminate, and often interminable, periods for what they *might* do. One might ask why the myth of their dangerousness persists and why we apparently feel a strong compulsion to lock them up. The answer would necessitate a book in itself. Probably much of it, however, revolves around our need to scapegoat another group (in this case, mental "patients") in order to shore up our own fragile egos. They are dangerous, we are not. They are "sick," we are not. The farther we put them away from us (a nice walled compound out in the country does very nicely), the easier it is for us to believe that they are fundamentally different from us. It is only when they intermingle with us that we see that they are not different, that their thoughts and their actions often mirror our own dark and irrational stirrings. Szasz provides a complete analysis of this in *The Manufacture of Madness,* where he contends that "... Institutional Psychiatry fulfills a basic human need—to validate the Self as good (normal) by invalidating the Other as evil (mentally ill)."[47]

This is illustrated by newspapermen every time a former mental "patient" commits a crime, especially a sensational one. Invariably, the fact of his former mental "illness" is reported as if it explained why the person did whatever he did. The studies reported above, showing that mental "patients" are *less* dangerous than the general population, are completely ignored because they do not correspond with what we want to believe. We want to believe that the person is "crazy," therefore not like us; therefore, he committed the crime. It makes life more comfortable if we can shore ourselves up with such little myths. The facts, however, are that you are much safer on the ward of any mental "hospital" at night than you are on the streets of New York.

The argument for mental "hospitals" that justifies them by saying that "patients" cannot take care of themselves is also specious. One study showed that of a group of mental "patients" who applied for admission to a mental "hospital" but were refused, 85 percent continued to function satisfactorily outside the hospital.[48] In another study, a mental "hospital" was reduced in population from 2,600 to 585 "patients" by finding alternative living arrangements in the community. A 2-year follow-up showed that 80 percent of them continued to function satisfactorily outside the "hospital."[49] And an analysis of the "patients" in another "hospital" found that 68 percent of them could be placed in community facilities if such were available.[50]

This is not to say that there are not large numbers of individuals who have moderate or severe problems in living, who are in need of a broad set of social supports, sheltered workshops, sources of income, and places to live. It only says that to label these individuals as "sick" and place them in a "hospital" is illogical, inaccurate, and a disservice to both the individuals and the community. Retreats, which will be discussed in Chapter 11, would be a better solution.

A final peculiarity of mental "hospitals" is that being in them can cause problems more severe than the problems which precipitated admission. This condition is called institutionalism and is characterized by extreme dependence on the institution and the loss of the ability to function outside it. Thus a chronic schizophrenic mental "patient" who sits on the back ward of a mental "hospital" and stares blankly at the wall hour after hour is as much a product of having been institutionalized as of having anything wrong with him. This is only now starting to be recognized.

The inevitable suspicion is that mental "hospitals" may even make people "sicker" the longer they stay. In a definitive study of this question, W. M. Mendel showed conclusively that the length of "hospitalization" had *no correlation* either with the percent of "patients" who were eventually able to return to the community or with the rate of readmissions. Furthermore—and much more damaging—he found that there was a *negative* correlation between the length of "hospitalization" and the "patient's" ability to function socially at work or in his family. In other words, the longer the "patient" is "hospitalized," the *less* able he is to function in society. Mendel summarizes his findings as follows: "The length of hospitalization had no effect on the quality or quantity of remission from the psychiatric disorganization...."[51] His staff, he says, "has recognized that no one has ever gotten well in a [mental] hospital...." *This* is certainly an institution worthy of discussion at the Mad Hatter's tea party.

6

Mental "Patients" as Not Responsible: The Fate of Jesus and Other Hippies

THE medical model is a kind of contract between a patient and society. And one of the important clauses in the contract states that the patient is not responsible for his disease. He may have been responsible for *getting* the disease—for instance, he may have purposely exposed himself to the mumps—but once the disease takes hold, he is no longer responsible. The fever, swollen neck, pain, and other symptoms of the disease are not thought to be under his control. They are, rather, part of the disease process itself.

In evolving the concept of mental "disease," psychiatry was obligated to include this clause of nonresponsibility. After all, who ever heard of a disease where the patient was responsible for his symptoms? The bylaws of the disease club would permit no deviation on this point.

At first it was easy. Psychiatrists pointed with pride to patients with brain tumors. Some such patients exhibit bizarre and irrational behavior—for instance, a man with a meningioma may begin swearing in the middle of a busy street for no apparent reason. This irrational behavior is due to the brain tumor and ceases when the tumor is removed. Such a man is not held responsible for his behavior; it is simply a symptom of his disease. Similarly, a person with typhoid fever is exonerated from responsibility for the strange things which he might say during a delirium. With such reasoning, the concept of nonresponsibility was firmly established as part of mental "disease," just as it had been for physical disease.

Doctor Frankenstein himself could not have done worse. The concept of nonresponsibility of mental "patients" has proven to be Pandora's box, which daily spews forth new evils—decreased self-esteem of those labeled as mentally "ill," the discrediting of their thoughts and achievements, the deprivation of their civil liberties, their involuntary confinement, and the use of insanity as a legal defense to excuse crime. Though originally applied for humanitarian reasons, the label "not responsible" has proven to be a millstone around the neck of those so labeled and often causes them to drown. It is a rose whose deadly thorns far exceed its lovely looks. Let us examine some of the thorns.

DECREASED ESTEEM

First, there is no question but that calling a person mentally "ill" is pejorative. Studies utilizing the semantic differential have shown that the public views mental "patients" as more worthless, dirty, dangerous, cold, insincere, unpredictable, and weaker than the general population. Another study showed that mental "patients" viewed themselves similarly as excitable, foolish, unsuccessful, slow, cruel, weak, curved, and ugly.[2] Thus the label decreases both the self-esteem of mental "patients" and their esteem by others. It makes them into a subhuman species. The only analogous situation in physical medicine is the label of leprosy.

Some have contended that the negative associations with the label mental "illness" are simply an unfortunate historical accident and that as we educate the public better they will disappear.[3] These people speak enthusiastically of the time when it will be no more derogatory to call someone mentally "ill" than it will be to say they have diabetes. This is unlikely. The pejorative connotations of mentally "ill" are inherent in the concept itself and are partly a function of the belief that these individuals are not responsible. As Theodore Sarbin summarizes it: "One can no more delete by fiat the evaluational component from 'mental illness' than eliminate the 'pleasantness' from the act of eating a preferred food."[4]

THE DISCREDITING OF OTHERS

A more serious consequence of the belief that mental "patients" are not responsible is the entry that it provides for discrediting others' thoughts and achievements. Since mental "patients" are not responsible, then everyone who can successfully be labeled as mentally "ill" can be ignored, depreciated, and even ridiculed. Their thoughts and their actions assume the same importance as those of a circus clown. This label, of course, then becomes a potentially deadly political and philosophical weapon.

It did not take long after the formal discipline of psychiatry began for professionals to begin using this weapon. Jesus was one of the first intended victims. Between 1905 and 1912 four books were published in an attempt to prove that Jesus was mentally "ill"—*Jesus Christ from the Standpoint of Psychiatry; Jesus: A Comparative Study of Psychopathology; The Insanity of Jesus;* and *Conclusions of a Psychiatrist.*[5] The authors focused on his ideas of grandiosity and persecution, ideas of reference, auditory and visual hallucinations, and fixed delusional system. If Jesus really was "insane," they imply, then all those things He did and said can be disregarded as the irresponsible ravings of a "madman." Other great figures in history and literature have been similarly subjected to this insidious pseudoscientific mudslinging—Copernicus, Galileo, Luther, Dostoyevsky, Nietzsche, and Kafka.

More recently, the label mentally "ill" has come into fashion politically. Psychiatrist Thomas Szasz has reviewed the case of Ezra Pound, accused by the United States government of treason during World War II. Instead of being brought to trial, however, he was labeled as mentally "ill" and incarcerated in a mental "hospital."[6] Any honest differences that Mr. Pound may have had with American policy were thereby glossed over and effectively shunted aside, since he was by definition not responsible.

Another contemporary example was the poll of psychiatrists taken by *Fact* magazine on the mental "health" of Mr. Barry Goldwater when he was a presidential candidate in 1964. Almost 1,200 psychiatrists judged him to be "psychologically unfit" in the poll, thereby casting doubt on his ability to hold office.[7] The United States government's persecution of former General Edwin Walker during his involvement in the civil rights struggle in the South is yet another example and a grossly irresponsible misuse of psychiatry. He was arrested, charged with sedition, and then committed against his will to a mental "hospital" for pretrial psychiatric examination. The effect was to discredit his political activity against integration. Szasz has documented this sorry case in detail.[8] The civil rights struggle produced abuses of psychiatry on the other side as well, as when civil rights workers were "hospitalized" for "observation" of possible mental "illness." As Robert Coles has noted, it was "a fashionable kind of slander."[9] The fact that both General Walker and civil rights workers could be discredited with the same weapon illustrates that it is a sword which can be used in the name of any and every political philosophy.

In recent years, there have been news reports that the Soviet government has adopted this same technique to discredit political dissidents. Poet Natalia Gorbanyevskaya, General Piotr Grigorenko, and biologist Zhores Medvedev, among others, have been detained on charges of "defaming the Soviet State," found to be "insane" by a panel of psychiatrists, and sent to mental "hospitals." This is a much more effective means of political suppression than simply sending them to labor camps in Siberia because it discredits everything they have said as well as removing them from circulation. Various groups within American psychiatry have censured the Soviet government's action and the collusion by Soviet psychiatrists. Most of the groups, very wisely, have included a condemnation of the practice in *all* countries, including our own.

It should be noted that society has a large stake in the use of psychiatry to discredit others. Insofar as I can call someone who disagrees with me "crazy," I can ignore the substance of his disagreements. What he says is irrelevant. The label reassures me that I am right—those who think otherwise have a "disease" of their mind and cannot think clearly. This ploy of self-justification is used commonly by individuals and, as has been pointed out, can be used by governments as well. If the idea of mental "illness" were abolished, this ploy would no longer be available; we would have to pay attention to some of our "crazy" critics rather than just cavalierly ignoring them.

It is also important to make a distinction between discrediting others by labeling them mentally "ill" and analyzing motivations behind another person's behavior, either public or private. The latter is not only legitimate but desirable. For historical figures, it has come to be known as psycho-history. The difference between the two is the difference between calling Van Gogh a schizophrenic or saying that he had private visions which influenced his painting. The first is a label which discredits him, the second a statement which tries to explain why he painted what he did.

DEPRIVATION OF CIVIL RIGHTS

Since a mentally "ill" person is not responsible, he cannot be thought of as a regular citizen. He belongs in an inferior class of beings who do not have the same rights, obligations, and privileges as people who are mentally "healthy." Laws vary in different states regarding which civil rights are abridged for the mentally "ill"; but usually included are the rights to vote, drive, make a contract, marry, be called for jury duty, and sometimes even stand trial. Depriving an individual of such rights is, of course, a gross violation of the Constitution and can only be done under the medical rationalization of the person being mentally "ill."

The deprivation of rights of mental "patients" has received little attention until recently and has usually been taken for granted. Those who have focused on it, however, have found that the facts are at variance with our assumptions and rationalizations. For instance, a mock election was held at the Bronx State Hospital in New York State simultaneous with the real gubernatorial election in 1966 and presidential election in 1968. The returns of the mental "patients" matched the returns from the Bronx as a whole almost exactly in their voting pattern.[10] One is left with only two possible conclusions: either the whole Bronx is mentally "ill" or there is no justification for the disenfranchisement of people whom we label as mentally "ill."

Another interesting study was one in which mental "patients" were used as jurors in a mock trial. Nine jury groups of six "patients" each were drawn from individuals labeled as "paranoids," "psychopaths," and "depressives" in a mental "hospital." Regular jurors from outside the "hospital" were used as controls. The results of the mock trial revealed that the "psychopaths" were most likely to find the defendant not guilty by reason of insanity; the "paranoids" were similar to the regular jurors in their findings; and the "depressives" reflected greater insight into the dynamics of the problems of the defendant than either the "paranoids," the "psychopaths," or the regular jurors.[11]

Further light is shed on the supposedly "crazy" thinking processes of mental "patients" by a study of attitudes toward death. Two groups of eighty-five "patients" and eighty-five "normals" were asked the following question: "If you could do only one more thing before dying, what would you choose to do?" The answers of the mental "patients" reflected significantly more social and religious preoccupations, e.g., "stop war if possible," "know more of God." The "normals," by contrast, answered more frequently that they would seek personal pleasure and gratification, e.g., "travel all over the world."[12] If anyone *has* to be deprived of rights, one wonders which of the two groups it would be more logical to deprive.

A very serious deprivation of rights is not allowing a person to stand trial. It directly violates the sixth amendment of the Constitution. Again it is the medical model which is invoked to justify such violations of basic rights. It would be unfair, it is reasoned, to require a person with pneumonia or a heart attack to stand trial. The person is permitted to get treatment for their disease first, then the trial may begin. So it is with people mentally "ill"—they should be treated first and then stand trial. Although it varies among states, the criterion usually used to determine whether a mentally "ill" person can stand trial is whether he can understand the charges against him, the nature and object of the proceedings and is able to assist counsel in his own defense.

This is another good example of the lovely rose with deadly thorns. The idea that a person can be mentally incompetent to stand trial opens up abuses of the grossest other—individuals incarcerated without a trial. In 1967, there were 15,000 persons either indefinitely committed on those grounds or being held pending determination of their competency.[13] This may be acceptable in an authoritarian state; but in a democracy, it should have been rejected in principle long ago.

At the Mattewan State Hospital in New York State, there were 200 individuals who had been waiting to stand trial for *over 20 years*.[14] Abuses of this label occur and have been well documented.[15] One recent study of individuals labeled "not competent to stand trial" showed that only 6 out of 501 people so labeled in Massachusetts were truly not competent.[16] The label has become a dumping ground for people whom the courts, for one reason or another, do not wish to bring to trial. In California, when the rules for civil commitment of mental patients were tightened (under the Lanterman-Petris-Short Act) the use of incompetency commitments increased six-fold.[17] It has also been shown that individuals committed to mental "hospitals" under incompetency proceedings are hospitalized longer than those who are committed civilly.[18] It can also be argued that "competence" is always a relative concept—a lawyer is more competent to defend himself than an uneducated laborer. Consequently, *every* instance of mental "illness" being used as an excuse for depriving a person of the right to trial is an abuse and should never be allowed to occur.

INVOLUNTARY CONFINEMENT

Among the most serious consequences of defining a person as not responsible is the power that then allows society to incarcerate him against his will. Such a person usually has broken no laws; but by acquiring the label mentally "ill," he becomes by definition not responsible, ergo, subject to detention and confinement. The medical model provides alternative rationalizations for the involuntary confinement of mental "patients"—that they are "infectious" like people with smallpox, or that they are dangerous like people with certain rare kinds of epilepsy—but it is the "not responsible" clause which is usually invoked when justification is necessary. A mentally "ill" person is said to be no more responsible than is a person in coma from a head injury and decisions regarding the necessity of "hospitalization" must therefore be made for both of them.

Involuntary confinement of mental "patients" is the rule, not the exception. Ninety percent of "patients" in American public mental hospitals are on committed status. This means that at any given time, there are approximately 350,000 persons being held on involuntary status in the mental "hospitals" of the United States. Although some of them are glad to be there, the point is that they do not have any choice. And not only may they be incarcerated, but measures of restraint may be used to keep them "under control"—including locked cells, strait jackets, and Mace.®[19]

The criteria for having a person involuntarily committed vary from state to state, but generally include dangerousness to self or to others. In some states, the criteria are very loose and vaguely worded; for instance, in Massachusetts, a person may be confined if psychiatrists testify that "he is likely to conduct himself in a manner which clearly violates the established laws, ordinances, conventions, or morals of the community."[20] This would include everybody I know!

The commitment proceedings themselves are a farce in most places. They are supposed to be civil proceedings in which evidence is presented by psychiatrists who have examined the "patient," the "patient" is given the opportunity to defend himself, and the judge then adjudicates the case. One might think that, since a person's liberty is at stake, such a decision would be made with a maximum amount of care and deliberation. In fact, the whole procedure is a monumental disgrace to the American psychiatric and legal professions.

There have been at least four separate studies of commitment proceedings. Each study was done by responsible investigators. The results are as follows:

Investigator	Number of Cases Screened	Average Time Court Spent on Each Case, min.	No. of "Patients" Represented by Legal Counsel
Scheff[21]	22	1.6	
Cohen[22]	40	1.9	0
Miller & Schwartz[23]	58	4.5	1
Maisel[24]	50	8-10	2

Incredible as it may seem, our judicial system is committing individuals to institutions—for indeterminate periods—on the basis of proceedings of just a few minutes' duration. Furthermore, this occurs not as an isolated event, but every working day in every state in the Union. Right now, 350,000 people are so confined. Can you imagine the outcry if this many people were being involuntarily confined for any other reason? But there is no outcry for these people—after all, they are *"crazy."* They really don't deserve the full benefit of our legal system! Better to save our valuable court time for people who have smoked marijuana and committed other such serious crimes. If this is justice in a democracy, then what is it like in a totalitarian state? Ivan Denisovich was given a fuller hearing before he was sent to Siberia.[25]

One can hypothesize that these short proceedings may have been justified if the court psychiatrists had carefully examined the "patients" prior to court. Sheff asked this question and found that the psychiatrists had spent an average of 9.2 minutes examining each case. Maisel also found that the examinations occupied only a few minutes and, in some cases, the psychiatrist had conducted *no examination at all* but merely relied on what nurses and others had written on observation sheets.

Maisel also makes the following observations about commitment proceedings:

> Patients were called by their first names, and when answering questions often were either interrupted by another question or else not listened to. Questions were so rapid-fire at times as to almost acquire a singsong or ritual-prayer rhythm.... One is further struck by the casual nature of the presentation of evidence. Whether "mental illness" or various kinds of deviant behavior are at issue, the judge commonly accepts, and even invites from those present, comments, allegations of fact, and judgments without attempting to verify these allegations or to substantiate charges which may play a crucial role in the final adjudication. Since the patient is often ignored and rarely has counsel, his ability to present counterevidence or argue effectively in his own defense is neutralized.[26]

And in the forty cases observed by Cohen, the court-appointed attorney never talked to any of the "patients" (*including* two who wrote him prior to the hearings), asked no questions of the doctors, did not study the court file, routinely signed the jury waiver form for each case, and collected $400 for his 75-minute attendance.[27] This ritual would qualify as low comedy were it not for the fact that individuals are being incarcerated for indeterminate periods in the process. It should be remembered that this whole sorry situation is made possible—indeed sponsored by—the medical model of human behavior. Born from the best of intentions, the present nightmarish situation is worthy of Kafka.

The consequences of involuntary, indeterminate commitment are well known. Every few weeks, the newspaper reports some person who has spent most of his life in a mental "hospital" because somebody forgot to determine when he got "well." For instance, a thirty-year-old man in 1905 stole a horse, a buggy, and harness. He was committed to a mental "hospital" as unable to stand trial and finally released 59 years later.[28] Another man was arrested as an attempted rape suspect and sent to a reformatory for a "sanity investigation." He was finally released 38 years later.[29] This must qualify in Guiness' *Book of World Records* as the most complete investigation in history! These examples could be multiplied by a list as indeterminately long as the sentences; and in the *Prisoners of Psychiatry,* lawyer Bruce Ennis describes a selection of such individuals in a "hospital" for the criminally "insane."[30] The impact of the book is to evoke horror in the reader—horror that such things still can take place in our society.

Less dramatic but more numerous than these newspaper cases are the thousands of individuals who, because they deviate from community norms of behavior, are labeled as mentally "ill" and committed involuntarily. The following case is illustrative:

> The mother of the petitioner—he is a 26-year-old, self-professed "hippie"—following an altercation with her son which resulted in his arrest, filed a petition that he be adjudged incompetent. Testimony at the sanity hearing held pursuant to the petition disclosed that during the past 8 years the man had been in and out of several universities. In addition to his beliefs in love and nonviolence, he professed to be an atheist. His beliefs and

personal conduct brought him into disagreeable conflict with his father as well as his mother and her husband. He fathered an illegitimate child, and resented the attitude of his mother and stepfather toward the child. Following the hearing and mental examination, the petitioner was declared incompetent and was committed. He appealed the court's determination.[31]

Fortunately, the court of appeals reversed this travesty of justice, deciding that the man's "strange behavior" did not necessarily indicate mental "disease." Individuals like this man can be found in many mental "hospitals."

The myth that mental "patients" are dangerous has been dispelled in the previous chapter and it cannot be used as a rationalization for involuntary confinement. As Szasz points out, a drunken driver is infinitely more dangerous to others than is a "paranoid schizophrenic," yet we allow most of the former to remain free while we incarcerate most of the latter.[32] It appears that we, who are psychiatrists and should know better, project our own irrational impulses onto others whom we cannot understand, label them as mentally "ill," confine them, and feel better. This is not to say that there are not individuals in every community who are dangerous to others, but they can be dealt with by a judicial system without pinioning them with a pejorative epithet.

Perhaps the most serious consequences of involuntary commitment have occurred in the Soviet Union. As mentioned previously, political dissidents have been incarcerated there by being labeled as mentally "ill," thus discrediting them (and their criticism of the Soviet government) and effectively removing them from society. It is the modern-day version of imprison-your-enemies, with the cooperation of a small number of Soviet psychiatrists.

The involuntary psychiatric incarceration of these individuals has been, and continues to be, a reprehensible act. But the really frightening thing about it is the sheer, compelling logic of it all, once the basic doctrine of involuntary confinement for mental "illness' has been accepted. A Soviet textbook on *Forensic Psychiatry*,[33] with contributions by G. V. Morozov, D. R. Lunts, and the other members of the staff of the notorious Serbsky Institute in Moscow, makes it clear that these doctors are not just facile tools of the Soviet secret police; they really *believe* in what they are doing and that it is part of psychiatry. After all, a person who writes tracts against the Soviet state, or hands out leaflets in Red Square, clearly *must* be crazy or he wouldn't do it. He has a delusion, which Morozov defines as "a rational judgment that does not conform to reality."[34] And since Marxist-Leninism is reality, as everyone knows, then the man is "sick," schizophrenic. Other symptoms which would confirm the diagnosis of schizophrenia are argumentativeness which is "a tendency toward unnecessary disputation and vacuous, fruitless casuistry."[35] In other words, the man disagrees with the party line and continues to verbalize his disagreements.

Now since psychiatrists hold the needs of the patient uppermost, the least they can do is remove him from danger to himself and others until he gets well. Since he is "sick," he is not responsible. And once labeled as schizophrenic, he may need care for a long time—even after he has gone into remission. According to Morozov:

> Remissions from schizophrenia with mild personality changes do occur. Patients in such a condition may also commit socially dangerous acts....However, since prolonged and persistent remissions without notable personality changes are comparatively rare, schizophrenics are usually adjudged not legally responsible during a period of remission.[36]

It would appear, then, that the psychiatric incarceration of dissidents in the Soviet Union can be rationalized by the psychiatrists as in the best interests of the "patients." The necessity to defend the Soviet state need not even be invoked (although elsewhere in the book it becomes clear that it can be, if necessary). All one needs is the doctrine of involuntary confinement for mental "illness" and a conception of the prevailing reality of that society. It is the logical, perhaps even the inevitable, outcome of the medical model of deviant human behavior.

And, as should be abundantly clear by now, such abuses need not be—indeed, are not—confined to the Soviet Union.

Psychiatric incarceration of dissidents can be used in any society in which the government is strong enough. And since it has the attractive feature of discrediting political opponents at the same time as it removes them from society, its use is inevitable as long as we view human behavior in terms of disease. In every developed country in the world, including our own, there is a Morozov and a Lunts waiting to do his psychiatric job if we will only give him a chance. This specter alone is enough to impel us to change our ideas about mental "illness."

THE INSANITY DEFENSE

The ultimate in the concept of nonresponsibility for mental "patients" is the insanity defense. It states that certain individuals who commit crimes while they are mentally "ill" are not guilty of the crimes and cannot be punished. They are "sick," therefore not responsible, therefore not guilty. This has spawned an imbroglio in courts of the Western world that qualifies as an official caucus race.

The literature on it is voluminous. Professor A. S. Goldstein, the author of one of the best analyses, claims that "for well over a century, the insanity defense has attracted more attention than any other issue in criminal law."[37] The whole subprofession of forensic psychiatry has grown up around it in an effort to clarify this interface between psychiatry and law.

It is important to note that the insanity defense is a product of the most worthy of intentions. It was partly motivated by a wish to humanize the penal system; by urging "treatment" rather than "punishment" of criminals, it has done much to fulfill its humanitarian heritage.[38] However, it is a sword which cuts both ways. As summarized by English social critic Barbara Wootton, "instead of treating lunatics as criminals, we now regard many criminals as lunatics."[39]

It should also be noted that the insanity defense serves a wide social purpose as well as its more restricted legal purpose. It gives us a mechanism for explaining some human behavior which we find difficult to understand. The motiveless murder—Raskolnikov's murder of his landlady in *Crime and Punishment*—makes us uneasy. If we can successfully label him as "sick," we feel reassured; for then he is not like us. This job of explaining unknown behavior formerly fell upon the clergy; psychiatrists have inherited it as they have inherited other aspects of the clerical role.[40]

The insanity defense dates back many centuries before formal psychiatry began. In the thirteenth century, it was known as the "wild beast test" in England (insofar as some individuals are like wild beasts, they cannot be held accountable).[41] In the sixteenth century, it was a central thesis in Johann Weyer's arguments that witches should be treated as "sick" rather than as criminals. In refuting these arguments, Jean Bodin commented at that time:

> If Weyer's sophisms and those of his wonderful doctors held good, the thieves and robbers might always appeal for mercy by blaming the devils for their deed; and since the officers of the law have no jurisdiction or power against the devils, one might as well cancel and erase all those divine and human laws which deal with the punishment of crimes.[42]

Four hundred years after Bodin pointed out this logical conclusion of the insanity defense, we have yet to learn it. We are, in fact, stuck at *exactly* the same point.

The legal precedent for insanity as a defense rests upon excusing individuals for crimes when they are committed by accident, in self-defense, or under duress. Thus, mental "illness" simply becomes another such excusing circumstance under which the person is not responsible and cannot be judged guilty.

The defense has three major variations. The McNaughton type (named after the man who shot Sir Robert Peel's secretary in 1843 and used in about two-thirds of the states) depends upon showing that the accused did not know "the nature and quality of the act he was doing or, if he did know it, that he did not know he was doing what was wrong." It is popularly referred to as the "right-or-wrong test." The second variety is the Durham Rule which was handed down by Judge David Bazelon in a 1954 case as a liberalization and broadening of the grounds for the insanity defense.[43] It states that a person is not guilty of a crime if the crime "was the product of mental disease or mental defect." It is called the "product test." The Durham Rule began to replace the McNaughton in a few states after its introduction. It led to such confusion, however, that in 1972 it was abandoned by a U.S. Court of Appeals in favor of a standard developed by the American Law Institute. This is a partial return to McNaughton and excuses a defendant if "as a result of a mental disease or defect, he lacks his substantial capacity to appreciate the wrongfulness of conduct or to conform his conduct to the requirements of the law."[44] Judge Bazelon, who both fathered the Durham Rule and also participated in its demise, contends that it never really had a chance because of the vagueness of psychiatric diagnoses and also the unwillingness of psychiatrists to admit their mortality.[45]

Given what has been pointed out about the nature of mental "diseases" in the preceding chapters, especially about their vague causation and diagnosis, it should be apparent that rules such as these can be extended with imagination to cover 100 percent of crimes. Every criminal can be fitted somewhere into the sprawling spectrum of behavior that has been incorporated as mental "illness." As such, their behavior will always be a *product* of their "disease" and there will always be a question whether they really *knew* "the nature and quality of the act." It should also be apparent, however, that judgment about whether a criminal act was a *product* of mental "disease," or whether the criminal *knew* right from wrong, will of necessity always be a subjective judgment. Although the psychiatrist takes the witness stand as a "scientist," he has nothing to offer the court on this matter except the same subjective evaluation of the criminal as any other man.

The consequences have been chaotic. For many years, we were spared the full effect of the storm because the McNaughton Rule was only used in cases where there had been flagrantly erratic behavior on the part of the criminal and everybody could agree that he must be mentally "ill." As psychiatry has come of age, however, and with the advent of the Durham Rule, we are now faced with the logical and inevitable extension of the insanity defense. In the District of Columbia, for instance, prior to 1954 about one percent of all criminal cases involved the use of the insanity defense. After

the Durham Rule was instituted, the percentage of cases in-
volving the insanity defense rose to 8.5 in 1960.[46] The only
reason why the insanity defense is not used more often is that
expert psychiatric testimony costs too much money for most
defendants and so the plea of "mentally incompetent to stand
trial" is adopted instead as easier and less expensive.

A widely publicized illustration of the insanity defense at
work was the case of Sirhan Sirhan.[47] The 60-day trial of this
man, accused of killing Senator Robert Kennedy, reached the
status of the theater of the absurd as the actors attempted to
ascertain Sirhan's sanity or lack of it. The assistant district attorney summarized it as a "venture into a quagmire."

Since Sirhan admitted the killing, the task for the prosecution was to show premeditation. This they did by introducing as evidence Sirhan's own notebooks in which he had
written specific threats against the Senator; the fact that Sirhan had gone target shooting at gun clubs immediately prior
to the crime; that he had told a man that he was going to kill
Kennedy; and that on the night of the killing, he had left a
firing range with a loaded revolver and gone to the hotel
where Kennedy was.

Undaunted by the facts, the defense set out to show that
Sirhan was mentally "ill" and therefore not guilty. They used
two psychiatrists and six psychologists to show that he had
been subjected to childhood traumas (bombings during the
1948 Arab-Israeli War), that he hated his father, that he was
a "paranoid schizophrenic," and that he had been in a self-
induced trance (assisted by the mirrors and lights in the hotel)
on the night of the killing. Psychological tests such as the
Rorschach ink blot test were introduced as supporting evidence. Their relevance to the case was summarized by the
prosecuting district attorney: "I think it would be a frightening thing for justice in this state to decide a case of this
magnitude on whether he (Sirhan) saw clowns playing patty-
cake or kicking each other in the shins in an ink blot test." To
refute this psychiatric testimony, the prosecution introduced a
psychiatrist of its own who confused matters still further by
claiming that Sirhan was not "sick" enough to be excused for
murder but was too "sick" to be executed.

The jury passed implicit judgment on the psychiatric testimony by finding Sirhan guilty. The press ridiculed the whole proceedings as "a psychiatric circus—maybe part of the clown act."[48] The fact is that the psychiatric testimony was introduced in good faith and is a logical, direct extension of the medical model. If there really are mental "diseases," then they must have causes. And the traumas of Sirhan's childhood certainly could be considered as sufficient causes. His behavior in killing Senator Kennedy then becomes a product of his mental "disease." Every criminal case can be looked at in this light. Given this muddle, the inevitable conclusion is that something is wrong with the basic model, the medical model of human behavior.

Another aspect of the case which suggests a very fundamental defect in the insanity defense is that the participating psychiatrists were considered to be among the most expert in the forensic psychiatry field. Doctor Bernard L. Diamond, the psychiatrist who introduced the tangle of mirrors, lights, and self-induced trances, is a professor of criminology, law, and psychiatry at the University of California. Less than one year before the Sirhan trial, he had been quoted as decrying the "quite worthless" quality of psychiatric testimony given in criminal courts and urged trial judges to "demand continuously better courtroom performances by the doctors."[49] If a man as aware as he was could fall victim to such a mishmash of pseudo-facts, then what hope is there that less experienced psychiatrists could fare better? It leads back inevitably to the conclusion that there is something very fundamentally wrong.

It is becoming increasingly clear that what is wrong is the whole insanity defense and, behind that, the whole concept of mental "illness." Each new well-publicized trial where psychiatrists take the stand and refute each other's testimony bears further witness to the fact that what they are discussing are values and subjective opinions, not bacteria and broken arms.

The trial of Garrett Trapnell, accused of hijacking a jet airliner in 1972, provides another useful illustration. Trapnell claimed that he had a "split personality" and that it was not he, but the other part of his personality, who hijacked the airplane. Therefore, he claimed, he was not guilty by reason of insanity. Helped by four psychiatrists who testified on his behalf, Trapnell succeeded in getting a hung jury. After the trial, he admitted that he had previously been arrested at least twenty times for major crimes but had spent less than 2 years in jail. On each occasion, he had invoked the "split personality" (which he had long since perfected), had been acquited on an insanity defense, and sent to a mental hospital from which he promptly escaped. He also admitted that his split personality was all a magnificent hoax.[50]

It is because of cases such as these that many people have concluded that the insanity defense should be assigned to perdition. Goldstein, quoted previously, calls for its total abolition.[51] Although he helped draft the law, he says that it has become "...a device for automatic commitment to mental institutions which may be worse than most prisons."[52] Karl Menninger would also throw psychiatrists out of the courtroom.[53] Seymour Halleck, a psychiatrist who has studied the issue extensively, sounds a similar note: "Medical involvement in issues of criminal responsibility is without a scientific basis, is socially impractical, and has probably done harm both to society and to the psychiatric profession."[54] And in 1973, President Nixon proposed legislation which would abolish the insanity defense in all federal courts because of its "unconscionable abuse by defendants."[55] This would be a constructive first step in the return of human responsibility—and human dignity—to man.

7

Mental "Disease" as Preventable: The Road to Psychiatric Fascism

THE most sacred shrine of the medical model is the temple of prevention. It is the sanctum sanctorum accorded homage equal to that given to cleanliness and godliness. The curing of a disease is good, but the prevention of a disease is always better—sixteen times better, in fact, since "an ounce of prevention is worth a pound of cure." Prevention is powerful, efficient, and American.

It began with John Snow's perspicacious observation on the London water supply in 1849; an epidemic of cholera was coming from somewhere but nobody knew where. Carefully Snow charted each case, then placed the data on a map of the city. The map revealed that all the cases were using the same water pump. Snow closed the pump, the epidemic was over, and the modern science of disease prevention was full-born.

Psychiatry lost no time incorporating the concept of disease prevention. In the first third of this century, prevention was the guiding force behind the "mental hygiene" movement. When the promises of this movement left its achievements far behind, it went into eclipse, only to emerge again in recent years as the "mental health" movement.

Advocates of preventive psychiatry maintain that mental "diseases," like typhoid and cholera, can be prevented. Insofar as mental "diseases" are like physical diseases, this is both logical and consistent. The causative agents of the mental "diseases" are transmitted from person to person or from the environment. Perhaps sexual problems, then, like gonorrhea, really come from toilet seats. As summarized by one observer: "Psychological and emotional pathogens are communicable. Their spread follows laws similar to those which govern the spread of biological pathogens."[1] Moreover, many psychiatric historians speak of "psychic endemics" at times when whole population groups become "infected" with the same mental "disease."[2] An example is the epidemic of "Dancing Mania" in the Middle Ages.

THE SCOPE OF PREVENTIVE PSYCHIATRY

One of the leading codifiers of preventive psychiatry has been Gerald Caplan. His definition of the field is as follows:

> Primary prevention is that preventive effort which is concerned with studying the population-wide patterns of forces influencing the lives of people in order to learn how to reduce the risk of mental disorder...[it] involves studying the provision of resources in a population and attempting to improve the situation when necessary—usually by modifying community-wide practices through changing laws, regulations, administrative patterns, or widespread values and attitudes.[3]

Caplan goes on to provide abundant illustrations of the scope of preventive psychiatry. Included are such areas of interest as Operation Headstart for an enriched preschool environment, an analysis of the amount of floor space per person in ghetto tenements, divorce laws, urban renewal, and visiting hours for parents on the pediatric wards of hospitals. Others have added family planning services,[4] the psychological assessment of police candidates,[5] and the content of car advertisements[6] as legitimate concerns for preventive psychiatry. In short, concludes Caplan, "the key factors which influence mental health in the community must be delineated in the areas of economics, politics, public health, religion, welfare, and education, to name a few."[7]

Caplan's views are widely shared by contemporary American psychiatry. The Group for the Advancement of Psychiatry issued a monograph in 1950 entitled "The Social Responsibility of Psychiatrists," favoring "the application of psychiatric principles to all those problems which have to do with family welfare, child rearing, child and adult education, social and economic factors which influence the community status of individuals and families, intergroup tensions, civil rights, and personal liberty."[8] Included under the last were problems of censorship and loyalty oaths; 4 years later, the organization published an entire symposium on this latter issue.[9]

More recently, this organization published a monograph entitled "The Dimensions of Community Psychiatry," extending the principles of preventive psychiatry to problems arising in institutional settings. Examples included "the rotation program in military service, the freshman orientation and counseling programs in colleges, the identification and removal of pathogenic leadership, and the modification of institutional routines and procedures with pathogenic effects."[10] Military psychiatrists may have to become involved over even a broader range, they maintain, including "acting as a participant or as collaborator on matters concerned with problems of morale, training, deployment, and command functions." This is preventive psychiatry.

It should be emphasized that behind this broad scope of preventive psychiatry lies the pristine logic of the medical model. Insofar as some human behaviors are really mental "diseases," and insofar as the causes of these "diseases" can be identified, then a psychiatrist has the right—indeed the obligation—to try and correct or remove these causes. It should also be evident from the above that a psychiatrist who hopes to carry out preventive psychiatry cannot be successful without becoming involved in the political process. Since he is dealing with social issues, and since social issues are decided politically, he must try to influence the political process. Politics and political action are logically inherent in the medical model of preventive psychiatry, a fact recognized by many observers.[11] Thus involvement in tenants' councils, cooperatives, minimum wage laws, and political campaigns are as valid for a preventive psychiatrist as are water purification and sewage disposal for a public health specialist.

The formal structures which have been created to accommodate the recent movement of psychiatry back toward prevention are the community mental health centers. The writings of Caplan, Lindemann, and the other "community psychiatrists" are, in fact, the cornerstone upon which the community mental health centers have been built. Since 1963 when this "bold new approach" was begun, almost 500 of these centers have been funded. Their mandate is not only to treat mental "patients" closer to home, but also to prevent mental "illness" by providing consultation and education to appropriate community agencies. If mental "diseases" really are like physical diseases, one would logically expect that if enough of these centers were established then mental "disease" might be completely eradicated.

Another example of an institution which has developed to do preventive psychiatry is the "Well-being Clinic." The theory is that people should be offered the chance for a routine check-up for mental "diseases" just as they are for physical diseases. At a clinic of this type in Montreal, the "original goals were to offer the ordinary citizen a routine, periodic check-up for his mental health, just as earlier established 'well-baby' and 'well-women' clinics offer routine physical health check-ups."[12]

THE PRACTICE OF PREVENTIVE PSYCHIATRY

Given sanction for such a broad range of activities, what does the preventive psychiatrist (or the community psychiatrist, as he is usually called) do in practice? It would appear from the above that he could legitimately do just about anything! In fact, the practice of preventive psychiatry is a subject of sharp debate and intensive concern among psychiatrists generally. One group has taken Caplan to heart and gone off in pursuit of the prevention of mental "illness." Their travels have quickly taken them to social institutions and the political process, with involvement in both. The rest of the psychiatrists have watched this with varying degrees of horror, now and then shouting "you just can't do that" or muttering "back to the hospital" as they reach for the reassurance of their stethoscopes.

The debate is really, of course, about the legitimacy of the medical model, although it only rarely gets translated into those terms. Until it does, it cannot be resolved. The community psychiatrists have logic on their side—the logic of preventing mental "disease." Furthermore, they can invoke the spirit of Hippocrates, an apparition which will speak in platitudes of prevention. Opponents of the community psychiatrists sense that something is fundamentally wrong, but are hard pressed to refute the logic of the medical model.

To illustrate the end-point of what a psychiatrist may do in the name of preventing disease, let us examine the work of Frantz Fanon. Fanon was a black born in 1925 in the French colony of Martinique. He studied medicine and psychiatry in France, then went to Algeria where he was baptized by the violence of the Algerian Revolution. What emerged was a revolutionary psychiatrist who saw the real problems of the world as racism and colonialism, not as intrapsychic conflicts related to Oedipus. He documented both very carefully with his psychiatric observations. In *Black Skins, White Masks*,[13] he eloquently describes the effects of racism; his observations have been corroborated many times but never surpassed. His *The Wretched of the Earth*[14] and *A Dying Colonialism*[15] quickly became basic primers for revolutionaries of the "Third World" and the "Black Power" movement. It was only Fanon's premature death from leukemia at the age of thirty-six that prevented him from seeing many of his ideas put into action.

For the "diseases" of racism and colonialism, Fanon prescribed violent revolution. This was the only medicine, in his opinion, which would be effective. The devastating effects of racism and colonialism are to reduce the individual's self-esteem to near zero. The only way it can be recouped is by the individual reaching out and taking it. It is not enough to have it given—for Fanon this is just more of "say thank you to the nice man."[16] The oppressed person must strike out and seize his self-esteem; only then will he be a whole person again.

Now anyone may disagree with Fanon's prescription for practical reasons, but it is difficult to disagree with his logic. The effects of racism have been documented too many times now and the effects of colonialism are being seen increasingly clearly. Both reduce people to nonpeople and shrivel up self-esteems like frost-bitten grapes. If increasing the self-esteem of a race or nation of people is the desired end point, then why not do it through revolution?[17] Fanon himself participated actively in the Algerian revolution and later tried to foment uprisings in other African countries.

Fanon frequently fell back onto the medical model to justify his thoughts and actions. And he never hesitated to use his position as a psychiatrist to gain his goals. Whether he really believed his own rhetoric about racism or colonialism being a "disease" is difficult to say. One biographer says that Fanon advocated social health as "...the first condition of mental health" and quotes a letter in which Fanon describes psychiatry as "...a medical technique for preventing man from feeling a stranger to his environment."[18] Another biographer agrees that Fanon perceived psychiatric problems in terms of the cultural and political environment.[19] Since his most important teacher was an expert in milieu "therapy," it is entirely possible that Fanon saw the Algerian Revolution as the largest milieu and group "therapy" project ever undertaken by man!

It is not the quality of Fanon's work which is in question. Indeed, he will probably go down in history as one of the major figures in the black liberation movement—the emancipation of black minds just as their bodies had been freed 100 years earlier. Nor is his logic in question, insofar as he justified his actions against racism and colonialism as preventing mental "disease." What is in question is the validity of mental "disease" itself. For once this basic concept is accepted, then one is led inevitably forward toward psychiatric fascism. Racism and colonialism no longer are social problems with tragic psychological consequences; they become *medical* problems. As exemplified by one observer: "Racism is one of America's major mental health problems. Concentrating on the elimination of racism is one of the first steps needed in America to improve mental health."[20]

Some may say that Fanon was an extremist and is not typical of true community psychiatrists. Perhaps Leonard Duhl and Robert Coles are more typical. Both are leaders in American psychiatry, both have made major contributions to social problems, and both have ultimately questioned the validity of the medical model. Duhl is a psychiatrist who, for several years, worked in Washington, D.C., for the Department of Health, Education, and Welfare and the Department of

Housing and Urban Development. While there, he used Caplan as a consultant. He has concentrated his attention on the plight of the inner cities and the many problems arising as they decay.[21]

Although Duhl has rejected the medical model as inadequate, he has at times used its terminology:

> The city ... is in pain. It has symptoms that cry out for relief. They are the symptoms of anger, violence, poverty, and hopelessness. If the city were a patient, it would seek help.... The totality of urban life is the only rational focus for concern with mental illness ... our problem now embraces all of society and we must examine every aspect of it to determine what is conducive to mental health.[22]

Duhl stops short of extending this metaphor to psychiatric solutions for the decaying cities, but such a step would certainly be logical. If the cities are breeding mental "illness," spray them with new programs just as if they are swamps breeding malaria. If the ghetto is the focus of an epidemic of mental "disease," close it up just as John Snow closed the London water pump. This would be the medical model of preventive psychiatry carried out in action.

A final example of a community psychiatrist is Robert Coles. His early studies were on the first black children who were integrated in Southern schools.[23] He then did studies on the Civil Rights Movement and more recently completed studies on migrant workers and other Americans. The recurring themes in his work are the effects of racism and poverty on people's mental "health." His descriptions of social injustices are brilliant.

Coles logically carries his beliefs into social action. Using the *New Republic* as a principal forum, he has exposed conditions of poverty in several states and demanded rectification by the politicians. For instance, his article on South Carolina ("Strom Thurmond Country: The Way It Is in South Carolina")[24] received national coverage in newspapers and resulted in such changes as the implementation of food stamps in the poverty-stricken area described.[25] Coles works as a psychiatrist, though he has repeatedly questioned the validity of the medical model for the problems with which he is concerned. "Must we," he asks at the end of *Children of Crisis,* "persist in applying rigid categories of 'sickness' and 'health' to social problems—and to people?"[26]

One might question whether there is enough knowledge of the relationship between ghettos, poverty, and mental "illness" for psychiatrists like these to become advocates of action. In fact, there is. It is known that people who are poor cannot purchase mental "health" services. So the work of these preventive psychiatrists cannot be dismissed simply as premature. They certainly know as much about the cause and effect relationship of these problems of mental "disease" as John Snow knew about bacteria, water, and cholera when he closed the London pump.

It is, of course, absurd to sanction and sanctify these social and political activities under the rubric of "disease" prevention. Fomenting revolution, lobbying for better housing, or urging greater availability of food stamps are simply not in the same category as purifying the water supply or building latrines. The former are attempts to solve social problems. Categorizing them as attempts to prevent "disease" simply muddies the water. When a concept like disease prevention is used to explain everything, it ends up by explaining nothing.

THE "PSYCHIATRIZATION" OF SOCIAL PROBLEMS

The idea of preventing mental "disease" can be criticized on grounds far more serious than those of semantics. For one thing, a psychiatrist has no training to do these things. For the first 9 years of his 12-year training course after high school, a psychiatrist receives the same training as a surgeon and a pediatrician. A knowledge of diseases of the body does not equip a person to solve social problems any more than knowledge of the blood supply of the uterus equips a person to teach sex education. Preventive psychiatry is defining more and more problems of human behavior as falling within its jurisdiction, yet its practitioners are unable to cope with what it already has.

Another criticism of preventive psychiatry, conceptualized as a medical specialty, is that it is impossible to evaluate what you are doing. A doctor can study the efficacy of penicillin for infections or surgery for gangrene, but he cannot judge the effects of a program of preventive psychiatry. Bloom has aptly summarized this:

> In a word, we are generally asked to evaluate the outcome of an undefined program having unspecified objectives on an often vaguely delineated recipient group whose level or variety of pathology is virtually impossible to assess, either before or after their exposure to the program.[27]

In another very perceptive paper, Bloom shows how the pregerm miasma theory of illness is much more closely analogous to what is presently occurring under the name of preventive psychiatry than is the medical model.[28]

Criticisms of preventive psychiatry as conceptually inadequate have become common. They have been aired both within and outside of the profession by such men as Burrows,[29] Bockoven,[30] Redlich and Pepper,[31] Szasz,[32] Leifer,[33] and Dunham. The last, for instance, suggests that "if a psychiatrist thinks that he can organize the community to move it toward a more healthy state, I suggest that he run for some public office."[34]

Preventive psychiatry can also be criticized on the grounds that the psychiatrization of social problems makes it *more* difficult to find real solutions to them. In contemporary language, it is a "cop-out," an abdication of society's responsibility by assigning social problems to the jurisdiction of well-meaning but naive psychiatrists. Once social pests are labeled and ensconced within the halls of medicine, then society can feel comfortable, not bothering to look for the real causes of the problems. The psychiatrization of the problems is mistaken for a solution. As Judge David Bazelon puts it: "When poverty, or racism, or crime is labeled a mental health problem, then society can defer to the experts for its solution, and everyone else is free to go on with business as usual."[35]

An example of a social problem which had become psychiatrized is that of abortion. Until recently, the decision as to whether an abortion was indicated was left in most cases up to psychiatrists. We in turn justified our decision by vague statements about the mental "health" of the woman. Often we would recommend an abortion on the grounds that the woman might commit suicide if the abortion was not performed, despite the lack of evidence that pregnant women with unwanted children commit suicide any more frequently than anybody else. It was all a sham, a shift of responsibility from society to psychiatrists. The more basic questions of who has ultimate jurisdiction over a woman's body, the interests of society, and the interests of the unwanted child were effectively shunted aside. The recent abortion reform is fortunately correcting this situation, taking the decision on abortions out of the hands of psychiatrists and putting it back where it belongs.

Alcoholism is another example. As long as it is classified as a mental "disease" then it is the doctors' (and specifically the psychiatrists') responsibility. Since up to 50 percent of arrests in most cities are for public intoxication, it is certainly in the best interests of the police to define this problem as belonging to someone else. Thus it is not surprising that such organizations as the Association of Police Chiefs and the American Bar Association have supported proposals to call all drunks "sick" and eliminate criminal penalties. If they are "sick," then it is up to the doctors to worry about why they drink, how to make them stop, and how to protect society from the drunken driver. Alcoholics may have abundant problems of living, but they are not "sick" in the commonly accepted sense of the word.

The issue of pornography is becoming increasingly psychiatrized. A recent newspaper article entitled "Smut Pouring Into City" warned that the mental "health" of the young people was being jeopardized by such "mental pollution."[36] The use of marijuana and other drugs is a problem which society is currently putting in the laps of psychiatrists. Even compulsive gambling is now being defined as a mental "disease" and thus a psychiatric problem; in England, psychiatrists are using electric shock "treatments" to condition the "patient" against gambling.

The incredible thing is that psychiatrists accept these problems as their legitimate "medical" concern. It is as if psychiatrists are all afflicted by some Eastern Mediterranean cross of *hubris* and *chutzpah*. Psychiatrists cannot possibly "cure" such problems as alcoholism or pornography or drug use. These are social problems, not diseases. This is not to say that behavioral scientists should not be concerned with these problems—they certainly should. But their concern should be with them as social problems, not as mental "diseases." The distinction is important and will be detailed later.

A major impetus behind this tendency to psychiatrize social problems arises from the vacuum of absolutes in our culture. This vacuum is associated with the decline of religious influence—the death of God, some claim. In the past, it has been religion which has supplied absolute values upon which we could base decisions. We were told that abortion was wrong, pornography was wrong, marijuana was wrong, gambling was wrong. There was no need to turn to psychiatry for solutions to such problems—you either did what was right or you went to hell. Life was simple. As religious influence has died, however, there has been a search for a new set of absolutes. Psychiatry has been willing to sanctify its values with the holy water of medicine and offer them up as the true faith of "Mental Health."[37] It is a false Messiah.

TODAY SCHIZOPHRENIA, TOMORROW THE WORLD

Certainly the most serious criticism which can be leveled at preventive psychiatry is that it leads logically to psychiatric fascism. If the problems referred to above are all really mental "diseases," then psychiatrists should be given increasing amounts of power so that these "diseases" can be "cured." Eventually they would be given control over almost every phase of human life and it would all be justified by the medical model. This is certainly not something that psychiatrists are consciously striving for, but rather a reasonable outgrowth of "community psychiatry." If cholera and typhoid can be controlled by requiring the building of sewers and the pasteurization of milk, then we must take whatever steps are necessary to control the "diseases" of racism and poverty. And individuals who are "infectious" and may spread a mental "disease" must be isolated in the same way a person with smallpox is isolated. As psychiatrist Lawrence Kubie points out:

Has a patient suffering from active pulmonary tuberculosis a right to spit in crowded public places? Has a
patient suffering from active venereal disease a right to
spread venereal disease until it becomes pandemic in
proportions? Has the patient with a sick mind a right to
spread filth and violence?[38]

The heavens cry out, No! No! No!.

We have not reached the millennium yet, but there are
signs that we are well along the path. Take, for example, the
case of the man who was caught exhibiting himself to a
young girl and was *sentenced* to 2 years of psychotherapy.[39] Or
take the recent legislation which was introduced in West Germany to classify mental "illness" with reportable diseases. In
other words, all "cases" of mental "illness" would be reported
to a central registry.[40] Eventually, it could be computerized
and you could get a print-out of everyone in the country with
such "diseases" as "homosexuality" or "inadequate personality." It is certainly logical—it's what is done for diseases like
leprosy and tuberculosis. Parenthetically, it should be pointed
out that the concept of community mental health (and its accompanying centers) has gotten off the ground very slowly in
Germany because, according to some of their psychiatrists,
there is an underlying fear that it heralds a return to the days
of national socialism and Hitler. Perhaps they know something we don't?

There are those who would urge us along this path even
faster than we are presently proceeding. Take, for example,
the views of G. Brock Chisholm, former Director-General of
the World Health Organization and President of the World
Federation for Mental Health:

If the race is to be freed from its crippling burden of
good and evil, it must be psychiatrists who take the original responsibility. . . . With the other human sciences, psychiatry must now decide what is to be the immediate
future of the human race. No one else can. And this is
the prime responsibility of psychiatry.[41]

It would appear that Plato's philosopher-king must become a

psychiatrist-king if this modest job description is to be fulfilled.

Another psychiatrist who can never be accused of being timid in his approach to preventive psychiatry is L. K. Frank. In his book *Society as the Patient,* Frank says: "There is a growing realization among thoughtful persons that our culture is sick, mentally disordered, and in need of treatment."[42]

And later in the book: "It might be suggested that the psychiatrist is uniquely competent to tell us how to practice the Christian injunction to love little children."[43]

Another approach to preventive psychiatry that can be called nothing less than fascism was suggested by psychiatrist Leopold Bellak. As a way to detect cases of mental "disease" early, in order to get them into treatment, Bellak offers:

> One way this approach could be introduced on a large enough scale would be to set up a network of metropolis-wide or country-wide central registries. There, the social, emotional, and medical histories of every citizen who had come to attention in any way because of emotional difficulties would be tabulated by computer. When these persons were divorced or widowed or encountered other difficulties, they could be offered guidance and treatment. These centers could also ensure quick referral to an appropriate therapist and a follow-up on the success of treatment.[44]

Bellak is aware that such a system might be interpreted as an infringement upon our civil liberties, but he has an answer to calm such fears:

> Some of my proposals may arouse violent reactions. For many, the suggestion of mental health legislation to control our lives in the areas we cherish most—freedom of thought and action—may invoke the image of Big Brother. And enforced treatment for emotional ills may cause the powers that be to fear brainwashing. But I am reminded that income taxes were once considered basic violations of personal freedom and fluoridation of water was held to be a subversive plot. If a Clean Meat Bill

and a Truth in Lending Act were finally enacted, why should a "Sound Mind Bill" be far behind?[45]

Why not indeed! Freedom of thought and action is a small price to pay for true mental "health." Doctor Bellak deserves to go down as the Mephistopheles of the mental "health" movement.

Yet another example to illustrate the logical conclusions of preventive psychiatry were the proposals submitted to President Nixon in 1970 by his former personal physician. These proposals urged psychiatric testing of all 6-year-olds in the United States to determine their future potential for criminal behavior. Those children who were found to be deviant and difficult to "treat" could be placed in "camps" for more intensive "treatment." Previously, this same doctor had proposed the testing of all high school and college students to detect mental "illness." Furthermore, a "mental health certificate" would be required of all young people as a prerequisite for any job of political responsibility.[46] This is, of course, no more than we require of food handlers who might have typhoid or tuberculosis.

As frightening as these proposals seem, it should be realized that they are the logical endpoint of preventive psychiatry when the medical model is taken as the starting point. As Bockoven points out:

> It would appear that, to be successful, a mental health program must first win acceptance of the view that the members of a community are to be regarded as patients (or potential patients) first and as citizens, second, and that the mental health professional should occupy the key position of coordinating community functions.[47]

A brilliant parody on this situation was published by Kenneth Keniston entitled "How Community Mental Health Stamped Out the Riots, 1968-78."[48] In it, he appoints General Westmoreland as the Secretary for International Mental Health and transforms the Department of Defense to the Department of Mental Health. For those "patients" who are difficult to "treat," he proposes a series of 247 Remote

Treatment Centers in the Rocky Mountains. As succinctly satirized by another observer of preventive psychiatry: "Today schizophrenia, tomorrow the world!"[49]

It should be added that there is no fascism where there are not people who are willing to abdicate their own liberties. So it is with preventive psychiatry. There are many who are willing to cede incredible power and authority to psychiatrists on the basis of their promise to "treat" these problems of mental "illness." The call of preventive psychiatry is the seductive call that offers answers for difficult questions, solutions for difficult problems. It is the call of the Sirens beckoning us toward the rocks.

Part II

The Neo-Educational Model

> The only time my education was interrupted was when I was in school.
>
> GEORGE BERNARD SHAW

8

On the Production of
Crap Detectors:
Education as It Should Be

ONCE upon a time there was a group of people called the Su who needed to go a long distance in order to survive. Since they had no transportation, and it was too far to walk, they began building vehicles. One group of Su, called the srotacude, built a large vehicle which would carry everyone; but there was one problem—it did not have any back wheels. Another group of Su, the stsirtaihcysp, built a small vehicle which could carry very few but which did have back wheels. When the Su fully realized the situation, there was a great outcry to take the back wheels from the smaller vehicle and put them on the larger vehicle. This, of course, meant that the smaller vehicle would have to be junked (which bothered only the stsirtaihcysp) but everyone would survive.

Faced with serious problems of human behavior, our situation is very similar to that of the Su. Psychiatry is one possible solution to the problems; but it helps very few people, is expensive, and will accept only those who call themselves "sick." Because it is inherently tied to the medical model, it leads, as we have seen, to all kinds of absurdities. In historical perspective, it was logical to try psychiatry as a solution; but now we can see that it inevitably carried us into a thicket of confusion and contradiction. Ultimately, it just does not work.

Education is another possible solution. It could provide help for everyone and is less expensive. Since it is not tied to the medical model, it does not demand that its recipients be "sick." The problem with education, however, is that it is missing two

115

critical pieces; and these pieces are currently attached to psychiatry. Without them education can go nowhere.

To propose education as a solution for problems of human behavior would seem, at first glance, like a fatuous thing to do. Education is currently discredited and undergoing a major upheaval. It is being attacked on all sides by those who claim that it is only producing "intellectual paraplegics."[1] It is portrayed as an intellectual desert, filled with drivel which is about as much attached to reality as tumbleweed. Teacher education is unrelated to the classroom and school administration is a paragon of the "Peter Principle." Worst of all is what occurs in the classroom itself. According to the 1970 Carnegie Commission report: "The banality and triviality of the curriculum in most schools has to be experienced to be believed."[2] How, then, can I possibly propose education as a solution for problems of human behavior when it cannot even teach people how to read?

The answer lies in the two missing pieces. I am proposing education not as it is, but as it would be if these two pieces were added. The proposed solution, then, should really be called neo-education rather than education as we know it. The missing pieces are behavioral science and the importance of the teacher's personality.

Behavioral science can be defined simply as *the study of human behavior*, both the behavior of other people and your own. Currently it is not an entity, but rather exists in small parcels in several disciplines. Psychiatry, psychology, psychoanalysis, anthropology, sociology, social work, political science, and several other disciplines each have part of it. The part held by psychiatry is a large one and, because you must become a medical doctor to gain access to it, is less available to the average person than the parts held by the other disciplines. Education was given virtually none of it and so it has had to build its curriculum on lesser fare.

The consequences of omitting the study of human behavior from education have been devastating. They are seen in the banality and triviality of its curriculum. They may also be seen in the revolt of contemporary students against it. No longer content to accept tradition as the guide, increasing numbers of students are asking for an education which has both social and individual relevance. They want to know why people behave as they do—both themselves and other people—and what the alternatives are. The indiscriminate devouring of mind-altering drugs and encounter groups may be seen as a measure of their hunger, for these avenues hold out the illusory promise of instant knowledge of the self. And given the curriculum offered by most educational institutions, a "joint" on the lawn at recess is very reasonable. You can lie there and take a quick trip around your mind, which is infinitely more interesting than anything taking place in the classroom. There are, of course, major exceptions to this generality—teachers who have smuggled some behavioral science back into the classroom—but they are pedagogical aberrations who stand out like skyscrapers in the middle of an educational desert.

The other missing piece of education is the importance of the teacher's personality. Though educators often pay lip-service to this idea, its real importance has been perceived only by psychologists, psychiatrists, and psychoanalysts within their respective fields. In the course of "psychotherapy," the personality of the "therapist" may play a crucial—even determining—role. Mental "health" professionals have evolved theories and coined words like "transference" to explain what was occurring. Since "psychotherapy" is really only a form of education about the self, it is not unexpected to find that the personality of the teacher also plays a crucial—even determining—role in education generally.

In spite of the fact that the importance of the "therapist's" personality has been known to mental health professionals for many years, they have yet to implement its implications. "Therapists"-to-be are not selected for graduate schools or psychiatric residencies on the basis of their personality characteristics but rather on the basis of their ability to memorize facts and achieve high grades. The results are predictable—intelligent yet often totally ineffective "therapists." And since the importance of the teacher's personality is hardly even recognized within the field of education, the results there are no better. Those good teachers who do exist achieve excellence in spite of, not because of, the system of selection and training. The major exceptions to these generalizations are psychologist Carl Rogers and his followers who have perceived the importance of personality and who have also tried to apply their findings to education; they will be discussed in detail in the next chapter.

Focusing on the teacher's personality brings a new dimension to the traditional idea of a teacher. In order to indicate this new dimension, I will use the word "tutor" in place of teacher. It is not a perfect word but it is preferable to coining a new word. It conveys a sense of teacher plus something more—the personality dimension. Tutor also includes the concept of being hired to instruct in a specific subject area (e.g., behavioral science), often on a private basis, and often not connected with an institution. As we shall see, all of these connotations are compatible with tutors under the educational model for human problems.

How Education Got Left Behind

A brief review of educational history will help explain how it got into its present dilemma. Up until 50 years ago, education was based upon the classical tenets of Plato, Aristotle, and Aquinas. The acceptable subject matter for the curriculum was what was "good for you"; this usually included Greek, Latin, mathematics, and handwriting. The role of the teacher was to set standards and see that they were met. Effective teachers were thought to be those who could judiciously mix admonitions with punishments; as such, teaching was a nice profession for frustrated policemen.

The advent of experimentalism in education, led by William James and John Dewey, shifted the focus to the student's motivation. The subject matter became incidental; the important thing was what the student was *interested* in learning, not what the curriculum contained. It was at just this time, moreover, that psychiatry, psychology, anthropology, and the other disciplines were dividing up human behavior for themselves. Education had neither the will nor the theory to fight for part of it because, according to the experimentalists, the content of the curriculum did not matter anyway. The failure of Dewey and James to focus on the importance of the curriculum is one of the chief limitations of their theories. They spawned an educational system rich in will but poor in substance, well-intentioned but eviscerated from birth.

Also under the influence of experimentalism, the role of the teacher shifted. Rather than simply being a policeman, the teacher now was supposed to facilitate the child's interests in whatever direction he chose to go. The definition of a good teacher was that of a good manager or administrator, facilitating the development of each child's interests and providing technical resources when needed. Even the idealists in the late nineteenth century, who gave rise to our teaching traditions in the humanities, saw the teacher as basically a plumber, drawing the truth out of student's minds in the manner of Socrates questioning the slave boy.

Just as the experimentalists did not realize the importance of the curriculum, neither did they perceive the importance of the teacher's personality. This is not surprising, since the roots of experimentalism lay deep within the idea of universal public education. Because education was becoming a right rather than a privilege, the concern was one of getting enough teachers for all students rather than what personality characteristics a teacher should have. Thus, although experimentalism had a profound influence on American education and continues to provide a major impetus for reform, it contains within its theories limitations which will prevent it from ever truly revitalizing education.

NEO-EDUCATION

The way out of the dilemma for education is to expropriate behavioral science and focus on the importance of the teacher's personality. As education now exists, it is bankrupt because disciplines like psychiatry absconded with the money. The death of psychiatry will make it easier for education to be revitalized; as long as psychiatry survives and hangs on to the two vitally needed pieces, education is not likely to go anywhere. It will continue to starve, because the real food is sequestered in cabinets to which it has no access.

Education has viewed its task too narrowly. A complete education should make man aware of the antecedents which predispose his choices as well as prepare him technically and

intellectually to carry out his choices. Intrapersonal and interpersonal knowledge is equally as valid an educational goal as
problem-solving ability, expressing oneself, and vocational
training. Such knowledge is essential to living in an increasingly complex society in which we have to learn why we do
what we do and how we interact with others. The purpose of
education must become, according to Postman and Weingartner's brilliant book on the subject, "... to help all students develop built-in, shockproof crap detectors as basic equipment
in their survival kits."'

In the future, we will have increasing leisure to contemplate ourselves and our relations with others. American society is evolving beyond a pure production phase and
entering a consumer phase. No longer is it necessary for everyone to just produce; we now have time to consume as well.
Yet our educational system remains mired at the earlier
phase and continues to turn out students who are experts in
producing everything from artichokes to zithers. Education
must allow us to learn how to eat the artichokes and play the
zithers as well as how to produce them.

In the final analysis, this broader view of education is more
compatible with individual freedom. The greater our understanding of the antecedents and constraints on our own behavior, the freer we are to explore new behavior. Education to date
has been used to prepare us for vocations which increase our
material freedom; perhaps now it should turn to education of
the self which would increase our behavioral freedom.

The Two Missing Pieces:
Behavioral Science and Tutors

ONCE behavioral science and the importance of the teacher's personality are added to education, it becomes a viable alternative to the medical model for problems of human behavior. There are logical reasons for including both additions within education and there are early signs of movement in that direction.

Behavioral science is long overdue to become part of the content of education. Learning about the self is intrinsically more interesting than learning about things. The study of people—their behavior, emotions, motivations, and limitations—has always intrigued students; but it has never been included in the curriculum. The result has been highly educated adults surreptitiously listening to "Portia Faces Life" and reading Ann Landers because these are the only places where people are the subject of discussion. Only a few of the wealthy have been able to study human behavior as a respectable subject; and to do so, they have had to define themselves as "sick" and pay $40 an hour to their therapist-teacher.

The recent generation of students has reflected this hunger even more blatantly. They have assigned much of the traditional educational content to concise four-letter categories; and in many instances, they have left the classroom altogether in search of something more "relevant." It is instructive to note that their wanderings almost inevitably lead up paths toward self-knowledge—experimentation with mind-altering drugs and encounter groups. It is the study of themselves and the study of others—human behavior—that "turns them on." If we listen to them, we can learn much about the shortcomings of what we have called education. And, of course, they are perfectly right—after a course on self-knowledge as taught by peyote, most of traditional educational curriculum looks pretty pale indeed.

For behavioral science to become part of the educational curriculum, not only must psychiatry die but several other behavioral science disciplines must die as well. The present study of human behavior has been artificially divided up and assigned to various nooks and crannies. Some of these are called psychiatry, psychology, social psychiatry, social psychology, psychoanalysis, child development, anthropology, ethology, sociology, and social work. In addition, fragments of behavioral science are often found in other disciplines such as political science, economics, and linguistics.

The present situation in the behavioral sciences is strikingly similar to that found among the Namnretsew, a large tribe living north of Tierra del Fuego. They are best known for their technology and their highly factionated society. The factions, interestingly enough, differ on the question of what is the true essence of an elephant. At last count, there were four major factions and innumerable minor ones. One of the factions, the stsigoloicos, climb trees to watch the pattern of elephant trails. The ways the elephants interact, they claim, is the essence. Another faction, the stsigoloporhtna, have made extensive studies of how elephants use bamboo shoots to cover their young. This kind of behavior, they claim, is the essence of the elephant. Still another faction, the stsigolohcysp, have argued that the only way to understand elephants is to study other animals; and they spend most of their time watching rodents on the jungle floor. Finally, the stsirtaihcysp faction argues that the essence of the elephant is inside him; and they spend hours looking inside elephants' ears with microscopes and minutely describing everything they see. The factions have become so hostile to each other that they have built high fences to keep the others out. Furthermore, it is said that each faction has developed its own sublanguage so that the others cannot understand. At last report, the factions had all started subdividing; and it was thought that the tribe was in danger of extinction because the elephants were being lost.

In order to develop an integrated and coherent science of human behavior to become part of the curriculum of classroom (and ongoing) education, then four of the major disciplines must merge. Psychiatry, psychology, anthropology, and sociology must take down their fences and synthesize their knowledge of human behavior into a unified whole. Instead of bickering about which of them has captured the essence of the elephant, they must become aware of how the "essences" are all part of the same animal. The only thing their disciplinary arguments have proven to date is the ignorance of those who engage in them.

Psychiatry, as we have seen previously, is a product of efforts at the turn of the century to make behavioral science into a medical specialty. These efforts succeeded in creating a formal discipline; but in the process, much valuable data on human behavior were locked up in the private offices of psychiatrists. The influence of early childhood experiences on behavior, for instance, is the almost exclusive domain of medical specialists called psychiatrists and psychoanalysts. If you want to learn what part of your own behavior is being determined by such antecedents, you must first call yourself "sick" and then contract with them to teach you. The tuition is very high.

Psychology, in contrast to psychiatry, grew into a discipline mostly by default. It began as the science of intelligence testing at the beginning of this century and was led by such men as Binet and Cattell. As psychiatry crystallized out as a pure medical specialty, psychology annexed a series of disparate segments of behavioral science that psychiatry was ignoring. Thus studies of normal growth and development (Gesell et al.) came to be included, as did studies of learning. The last was an especially ironical addition to psychology since the basic Pavlovian theories upon which learning psychology is founded are neurophysiological—straight from the basic sciences of medicine. If any segment of behavioral science should have been categorized under medicine, then logically this should have been one of the first. But logic was not part of the distribution process, so learning theories became the backbone of clinical psychology.

During World War II, psychology broadened itself from being primarily concerned with rats and mice to include people. The severe manpower shortages of psychiatrists led to the utilization of psychologists to "treat" people. From that point on, clinical psychology has grown to challenge the experimental psychologists for leadership of the discipline.

Psychology might have been expected to become *the* science of human behavior but it did not. Rather than broaden its purview to include psychiatric, anthropological, and sociological concepts, it instead retrenched itself with even higher fences. As seen by psychologist Carl Rogers today: "Academic psychology is, I think, leading every field in dogmatism, rigidity, narrow orthodoxy, and scorn of social involvement."[1]

It should be said that psychology never really had a chance to become *the* science of human behavior. From the beginning, it has existed as the handmaiden of psychiatry, told by its bigger brother what it could do or not do. Whenever this relationship has been challenged, psychiatry has invoked the medical model to reinforce its authority: "We are doctors, so we know best what you should be doing or not doing." And all too often psychology has meekly submitted to its imperious sibling and accepted its role as second-class citizen.

It is no wonder, then, that even though psychology became part of the classroom curriculum (at the college level), it has not satisfied the thirst for behavioral science. Students in the last two decades flocked to its table, as they are now flocking to anthropology and sociology. The only things they found on the menu, however, were rats á la maze and overcooked cognitive processes as prepared by Piaget. Essences were everywhere to be found, but the elephant was gone.

Simultaneous with the rise of psychiatry and psychology as disciplines were the emergence of anthropology and sociology. The former has its roots in the nineteenth century studies of "primitive society" by such men as Tyler, Morgan, and Frazier. It continued to be a rather esoteric pursuit of strange customs well into this century. A practical turning point was

Ruth Benedict's study of the Japanese character during World War II, *The Chrysanthemum and the Sword.* For the first time, it became clear that understanding other cultures might have some practical benefits.

However, the narrow base which it inherited has prevented anthropology from becoming *the* behavioral science. Its journals and meetings abound with superficial aspects of human behavior, as if mannikins and not people were being studied. Picking up a recent edition of the *American Anthropologist,* for instance, I find such earth-shaking articles as "Spheres of Influence in Aughnaboy" and "Kujaama: Symbolic Separation Among the Diola-Fogny."[2] Also in this issue is the continuation of a discussion on the nutritional value of regular cannabalism versus irregular cannabalism in case I want to know the amount of protein available in the flesh of a 120-pound man. In anthropology, elements of motivation or emotion are missing, segmented off into psychology and psychiatry and not considered "proper subjects" for true anthropologists. Despite such shortcomings, anthropology has become increasingly attractive to students at the college level who are trying to find courses that are "relevant."

Sociology grew out of the same nineteenth-century tradition as anthropology but has gone off into an even narrower corner. From the work of men like Spencer and Durkheim arose theories of how man behaves not as an individual but as a member of a social group. The influence of the group on human behavior then became reified as the essence of human behavior and sociology was born. Although several sociologists and psychologists have tried to bring the individual back into the equation (e.g., Robert Merton and Kurt Lewin), the sociological discipline remains a relatively sterile field without data from the other behavioral sciences.

A true behavioral science, of course, would not be confined to the data from these four disciplines. Though the merging of these four would provide an excellent beginning, other pieces would have to be brought in as well. The knowledge from biology regarding our inherited predispositions must be included. Just as the house cat and the family dog still hunt although well fed, man carries with him physiological and chemical responses (e.g., the fight-or-flight instinct) which in part determine his behavior. Similarly, we must include knowledge from areas like ethnology and comparative animal behavior. What can we learn about creativity, for instance, from watching chimpanzees who when allowed to paint pictures throw tantrums when their paint and brushes are taken from them before their picture is finished?[3] Presently knowledge such as this is sequestered off in obscure corners frequented only by biologists.

When all of this knowledge of human behavior is mixed together without disciplinary boundaries, then a true behavioral science becomes possible. It could be taught at all levels, both formally and as continuing education. It could be taught in the classroom as well as individually by a tutor. People would learn about themselves as part of their general education and they could take as many "advanced courses" on it as they wanted.

The skeptic will immediately say that such a scheme is impossible for there is too much knowledge for everyone to know. To try to produce a true behavioral scientist, he will argue, would be to overwhelm a person with information. I agree that everyone cannot know everything about human behavior. Therefore, there will have to be some division of the information.

One possible division would be totally different from the present one. The disciplinary divisions of psychiatry, psychology, anthropology, and sociology are divisions drawn along the lines of antecedents of human behavior. For instance, if you study the childhood experiences leading to aggressive behavior, you are a psychiatrist; if you study how aggression is learned in rats, you are a psychologist; if you study aggressive behavior among a South American tribe, you are an anthropologist; and if you study aggressive behavior among groups in our society, you are a sociologist.

A more logical way of dividing behavioral science knowledge would be by kinds of behavior. Thus, in the example given above, a behavioral scientist might become an expert in aggressive behavior, encompassing all the antecedents and manifestations of such behavior. Other behavioral scientists might become experts in sexual behavior, communicative behavior, acquisitive behavior, loving behavior, the behavior of self-denial, and so on. Such an expert would try to understand all aspects of the behavior from the most common expressions of it to its extreme examples. It is another way to slice the pie of knowledge.

Previous Attempts to Bring Behavioral Science to Education

There have been some attempts to bring behavioral science to education and such attempts have become increasingly common. Almost every school system and every graduate department of education has one or two individuals who are doing it; more often than not, however, such individuals are regarded as introducing "frivolous" subject matter and are tolerated by their colleagues with only thinly veiled contempt.

In primary and secondary schools, these people are most likely to be teachers of social studies or home economics. The former has become increasingly people-oriented in recent years, with infusions from anthropology and sociology. The latter occasionally leads to significant discussions about interpersonal relationships. Since there are few teachers who have the courage or ability to allow talk to stray too far in this direction, however, home economics often stops at the mechanics of running a house. It is a telling commentary on our civilization that more time is spent teaching how to make bread than is spent teaching how to make a marriage.

School guidance counselors are another potential source of behavioral science in the schools. Too often, however, they become linked to vocational guidance and testing alone. Classroom teachers send students with problems to be tested and counseled rather than recognizing that the problems may well be shared by most or all members of the class.

Mental health professionals themselves have occasionally become involved with education. One example is Anna Freud, whose *Introduction to Psychoanalysis for Teachers*[4] was written in 1930. This book says nothing about teaching psychodynamics to children; rather it tries to teach teachers so that they may understand the children and themselves.

The book was popular in the 1930s, during the period when psychoanalysis was popular among educators. At all times, however, it is made clear that psychoanalysis is something brought to education from outside, like the missionaries bringing the gospel; at no time are its principles actually synthesized with education to be used by students.

Variants on this form of mental "hygiene" have emphasized the importance of the teacher in the early diagnosis of mental disorders in children (e.g., Gerald Caplan's work) and the role of the school in actually treating disturbed children. A good example of the latter is Summerhill, a well-known private school in England. In describing what occurs there, Erich Fromm says the school "mixes education with therapy."[5] This school-is-therapy approach also dominates the report of the Joint Commission on Mental Illness and Health called the *Role of Schools in Mental Health*.[6] The emphasis is on how schools can help mental health professionals do their job; there is no exploration of any real synthesis between psychiatry and education.

Another variant of mental "hygiene" in schools is a group of "mental hygiene environmentalists." This group strives to create a mentally "healthy" classroom, whatever that is supposed to be. They describe their goal with drivel such as the following:

> The school should introduce the child to his environment and help him get on closer terms with it. He will feel more assured and less overwhelmed with the complexity of today's living. Miss Williams' room is a busy workshop; the children are learning and know that they are. Their step is springy. "I'm getting to know you, old world!" they seem to say.[7]

An occasional psychoanalyst has moved in the direction of an educational model for therapy, but such movements always stop short of any real synthesis. Lawrence Kubie, for example, deplores the sterility of education when self-knowledge is not included:

> Can there be wisdom even about the objective world around us in the absence of wisdom about the world

within.... Without it we can have no adults but only aging children armed with words, paint, clay, and atomic weapons, none of which they understand.[8]

But when Kubie reaches for a prescription to cure this educational malaise, he specifically rejects the synthesis of education and "psychotherapy." He does not seem to connect the fact that education is naked precisely because psychiatry, as one of the behavioral sciences, is wearing most of the clothes.

There is another group, the educational psychologists, who might have been expected to explore the interface between education and behavioral science. This is especially so since the two leaders of the progressive movement in modern education, John Dewey and William James, published textbooks of psychology within 3 years of each other before the turn of the century. What more promising start could be hoped for?

The promise was never kept. As the separate behavioral science disciplines emerged and strengthened themselves, each cut off a segment of human behavior and went off in a corner to play with it. Educational psychology took only the physiological aspects of the learning process, a rather sterile field when compartmentalized by itself. Learning was studied by watching rats in a maze—instincts, reflexes, growth, physical structure, conditioning, laws of learning, and so on. No emphasis was placed on the fact that a man differs fundamentally from a rat in that he can learn about himself! He can look at his *own* instincts and reflexes as well as study them in other species. Furthermore, the educational psychologists have paid practically no attention to the dimensions and importance of the teacher-student relationship. Finally, by exclusively focusing on the process of learning, the educational psychologists have failed to stress the importance of content: people will learn only what they perceive is worth learning. For all of these reasons, educational psychology has never worked toward any real synthesis of behavioral science and education; it became trapped between its own stimulus and response.

A handful of diverse individuals, however, have really moved toward such a synthesis in either theory or practice. To date, they have been too few to have had any significant impact on the educational or behavioral science establishments; consequently, their efforts have often sparked once and gone out.

An example of a theorist in this group is psychiatrist Thomas Szasz. In his *Ethics of Psychoanalysis*,[9] he begins to explore the implications of calling "psychotherapy" education. Regrettably, he has never fully developed this line of thought. Another theorist is British educator John Wilson; his *Education and the Concept of Mental Health*[10] questions the whole idea of mental "health" and sees problems as rather caused by "mislearning." Psychologist Richard Jones also called for a synthesis of "psychotherapy" and education in his *Fantasy and Feeling in Education*.[11] The big stumbling block, according to Jones, is that the medical model forces one to define all students as "patients."

Perhaps the most promising attempts to introduce behavioral science into education have originated in the humanistic psychology movement. Encouraged by pioneer leaders like Carl Rogers and Abraham Maslow, an increasing number of humanistic psychologists have turned their attention to the classroom. Schools of education such as those at the University of Massachusetts under Dwight Allen[12] and the University of California at Santa Barbara under George Brown[13] have made these attempts respectable within the educational community.

There are limitations to the movement, however. First, the humanistic psychologists are not bringing all of behavioral science to education but only the psychology portion. It is as if they got on the right train but brought only one of several pieces of luggage that they will need for the trip. Anthropology, sociology, psychoanalysis, and the others were left on the platform. It may also be questioned whether the dichotomy between cognitive and affective education so strongly stressed by humanistic psychologists[14] is a valid one. Getting in touch with one's feelings is part of behavioral science, but feelings can be studied cognitively as well. By stressing the encounter-group-in-the-classroom too strongly, there is the danger of scaring away many students who are prepared to study other people's feelings objectively but are not yet prepared to study their own feelings subjectively.

Humanistic psychology has also been impeded by being confused with the free-school movement and unstructured education generally. This is because many humanistic psychologists have supported the movement. It should be noted, however, that there is no necessary relationship between the two; one may postulate the importance of personality characteristics of the teacher in a structured classroom as well as in an unstructured classroom. It will be too bad if the valuable lessons which humanistic psychologists have to teach education are lost in the din of the free school. Finally, humanistic psychologists have been slow to be accepted by some of their colleagues because of their missionary zeal. By presenting their doctrines as the most important news since the Sermon on the Mount, and dealing with those who oppose them with the tolerance of a twelfth-century crusader, humanistic psychologists have often alienated their friends and armed their enemies.

The few times when the concepts of behavioral science have actually been introduced into the classroom have been almost uniformly successful. This introduction has occurred either as separate course, as behavioral science units in existing courses, or as informal sensitivity-type verbal exploration. Three examples of the first are summarized in a 1951 report from the Group for Advancement of Psychiatry.[15] In the Forest Hill Village Project in Toronto, for example, a "human relations class" was offered to classes 4 through 12.[16] More recent examples are Roen's work teaching behavioral science to fourth graders[17] and Bruner's course, "Man—A Course of Study."[18]

The integration of behavioral science into existing courses was attempted by Ojemann in Iowa. As evaluated by visiting psychiatrists, "the object is to inculcate certain principles of psychodynamics so that they are always ready for application in daily life, much in the same manner that a child who knows arithmetic will be able to apply his knowledge for all the ordinary daily requirements in the use of numbers."[19] Finally, the introduction of behavioral science through informal sensitivity-type verbal exploration has been carried out successfully in many schools. Ongoing attempts to introduce behavioral science into the classroom are summarized in *People Watching,* a publication begun in 1971 and dedicated to the idea "...that since children are human beings too, they might enjoy studying about themselves and others."[20]

For older students, there have been sporadic attempts to

introduce integrated behavioral science teaching at the college and university level. The Harvard program in social relations was an example. Unfortunately, the experiment failed because it merely juxtaposed traditional behavioral science disciplines under a common roof rather than actually integrating them. A true synthesis will not occur until the boundaries are erased. Medical schools have also begun such juxtapositions (e.g., departments of psychiatry and behavioral science) but also with little true integration.

Also interesting are isolated attempts to center learning around specific problems. Manhattan College's program in "peace studies" is such an effort; the student is expected to learn about the biology of human aggression, intergroup conflict, arbitration and mediation, the history of peacemaking, and the literature on peace. By beginning with a problem such as this, it is possible to cut across a multitude of traditional disciplines and become a true expert on the problem. Most colleges, however, have such rigid departmental boundaries that it would be going against the grain and therefore difficult to carry out. For this reason, it may be easier to make innovations like this in institutions not connected with a college or university; an example is the Western Behavioral Science Institute in La Jolla, California, which was founded as a nonprofit organization to develop a united behavioral science with practical applications for human problems.

It should be noted that many of the leading figures in the behavioral sciences, both current and in the recent past, have been looked upon as leaders precisely *because* their work has encompassed more than a single behavioral science discipline. Such leaders develop beyond being only a psychiatrist, psychologist, anthropologist, political scientist, or whatever and achieve higher stature as a generic behavioral scientist. Examples of such individuals are Henry Murray, Kenneth Boulding, René Dubos, Jerome Frank, Harold Lasswell, and Harry Stack Sullivan.

The "Science" of Behavioral Science

A brief word should be said about the "science" half of the behavioral science term. What do we mean by designating it as a science? To call something a science today is as much evaluative as it is an indication of methodology. Science means goodness, purity, efficiency, reliability, fidelity, and even American patriotism. Everything claims to be based upon science if it hopes to be accepted. This in itself is sufficient reason to call it "behavioral science."

It is also justified to call it "science" in terms of methodology. The scientific method includes observation, experimentation, logical reasoning, and measurement, all of which are compatible with the science of human behavior. It must not be supposed, however, that behavioral science follows laws as closely as physical science. The farther you move away from things and toward people, the less precise the scientific method necessarily becomes. Thus Newton's falling apple obeys laws precisely (the physical sciences), a growing tumor of the lung obeys laws less precisely (the medical sciences), and human behavior obeys laws still less precisely (the behavioral sciences). The farther away from the apple you move, the more causation increases from a single cause (gravity on the apple) to many causes. Furthermore, human beings have the perverse attribute of being able to contemplate their own actions, unlike apples. Thus if you predict John will hit Peter in a given situation, he may not do it just because you predicted he would. And if you predict he will not hit him because you had predicted he would, then he may hit you instead. So the human factor considerably modifies classical concepts of what is "science."

THE EVIDENCE FOR USING TUTORS

The importance of the teacher's personality is the other factor missing from the educational equation. There is evidence that it should be added if we hope to emerge with the correct answer.

Almost all the evidence emanates from Carl Rogers' work, both his own and that which he has inspired. Rogers himself argues that a "therapist" or teacher cannot *teach* anything significant to anybody; rather, all a "therapist" or teacher can do is provide conditions under which a person can learn. Anything that can actually be taught, he contends, "...is relatively inconsequential, and has little or no significant influence on behavior."[21] An example of this is the names of the capital cities for each state; it can be taught, but it is inconsequential for the person. Significant learning, on the other hand, is what the person *learns,* not what he is taught:

> By significant learning I mean learning which is more than an accumulation of facts. It is learning which makes a difference—in the individual's behavior, in the course of action he chooses in the future, in his attitudes and in his personality. It is pervasive learning which is not just an accretion of knowledge, but which interpenetrates with every portion of his existence.[22]

The conditions which the "therapist" or teacher must provide in order for significant learning to take place are conditions inherent in the personality of the "therapist" or teacher; these are genuineness (or authenticity), empathy, and unconditional positive regard. The "therapist" or teacher must share himself genuinely (rather than playing a role), empathize (rather than remaining aloof), and like and respect the person who is seeking help. Rogers sees good "therapists" and teachers as interchangeable and believes that the same basic process occurs in both cases.

There is abundant evidence to back up this theory. In "psychotherapy," a series of experiments have been done contrasting "therapists" having Rogerian personality characteristics with those who do not have them. The former get significantly better results with "patients" than do the latter; much of this work has been summarized by Truax and Carkhuff.[23]

Psychoanalytic and behavioral type "psychotherapies" have not taken personality characteristics of the "therapist" into serious consideration until recently. Following the lead of Rogerian "therapists," this is now in the process of changing. Increasingly commonly among psychoanalysts, the point is made that the particular personality characteristics of a given psychoanalyst either assist him or impede him with particular kinds of "patients." Moreover, the analytic contribution of the theories of transference and countertransference between "therapists" and "patients" suggests the real dimensions of what may occur in the learning process.

Among behaviorists too, there has been an increasing awareness of the importance of the "therapists' " personality. Although behaviorists in theory achieve "patient" improvement exclusively through their technique, it may be that the personality of the "therapist" plays a much greater role than has previously been suspected. One observer of Dr. Joseph Wolpe, one of the best known behaviorists, found that he has all the personality characteristics deemed essential by Rogers, Truax et al.:

> Dr. Wolpe is a warm, soft-spoken, pleasant man. He is polite, shows great interest in his patients, answers all their questions thoughtfully, allows no anxiety-producing silences, and approaches each pati nt enthusiastically. His questions are framed in an egosyntonic way. No strict demands are made on the patient, nor is he admonished in any way. Those in attendance frequently remark about how easy it is to talk with Dr. Wolpe and how relaxed they feel while watching him do therapy. Truax's attributes of the effective psychotherapist seem very much in evidence with Dr. Wolpe.[24]

Observations such as these are equally as applicable to education as they are to "psychotherapy." Rogers' *Client-Centered Therapy* contains a chapter entitled "Student-Centered Teaching," in which he says:

> If the creation of an atmosphere of acceptance, understanding, and respect is the most effective basis for facilitating the learning which is called therapy, then might it not be the basis for the learning which is called education?[25]

Rogers has reviewed the research evidence showing that effective teachers (as measured both by their superiors and their students) have higher levels of the personality characteristics which he considers crucial.[26]

Other experiments also corroborate this. In one study, 120 third-graders were monitored on how fast they learned to read. Their eight teachers were assessed for the qualities of genuineness, empathy, and nonpossessive warmth. It was shown that the children clearly learned to read faster under the teachers who offered higher levels of these three qualities.[27] In another study, first-graders were found to improve on intelligence tests and self-concept as their teachers improved in interpersonal skills.[28] When teachers listen to their students rather than lecture to them, the students get better grades and learn more. In a comprehensive review of all the evidence available for this, D. N. Aspy concludes that "...a teacher's increased positive regard for students is translated into classroom behavior which elicits higher levels of cognitive functioning from the students."[29] In other words, what the teacher thinks about the student and how the teacher relates to the student will determine what the student learns.

Another study which points in the same direction was done on the ideal teacher-student relationship. The researchers took data which had been collected by Fiedler on the ideal "therapist-patient" relationship and just changed the words to "teacher" and "student." They then had forty-one teachers sort the data in the same way as Fiedler had had "therapists" do. The results were the same and led the authors of the report to conclude that "...there are common characteristics in good helping relationships wherever they are found and whatever the technique and roles that may be involved."[30]

Further work by Combs and his colleagues at the University of Florida showed that people considered to be high performers in any of the helping professions (counselors, teachers, ministers, nurses) were very similar to each other in their beliefs about themselves and other people. As compared with low performers in these professions, the high performers saw other people as more adequate, trustworthy, wanted, self-revealing, and involved.[31] All of these studies can be summarized by Rogers' observation:

> So we can say, with a certain degree of assurance, that the attitudes I have endeavored to describe are not only effective in facilitating a deeper learning and understanding of self in a relationship such as psychotherapy, but that these attitudes characterize teachers who are regarded as effective teachers, and that the students of these teachers learn more, even of a conventional cur-

riculum, than do students of teachers who are lacking in these attitudes.[32]

A common thread running through these studies is the implication that the *relationship* between the teacher and the student is the crucial variable. Teachers who become involved with their students, who share themselves, and who assume the dignity and worth of the child get the best results. As one observer describes it: "Then there is mutuality, a sense of joint participation in life. It is very much like the joint creation of a poem, or painting, or symphony. Each person affects the other person in the creation."[33]

This corresponds closely with my personal experience as a "psychotherapist"; those "patients" whom I respected and became involved with appeared to "get well" (show significant changes in behavior) during the course of "therapy" and I, too, was affected. Conversely, those "patients" whom I did not respect showed little change. Not coincidentally, William Glasser, a psychiatrist who claims that his "reality therapy" works equally well in the classroom as in his office, advocates an intense personal involvement between the "therapist" and the "patient."[34] Both "psychotherapy" and classroom learning, then, appear to be part of a larger and more inclusive category of personal relationships—interpersonal learning.

A final aspect of the relationship between teachers and students (and also between "therapists" and "patients") is that students learn more if the teacher expects them to. This has been shown repeatedly in controlled experiments and has been referred to as the Pygmalion effect.[35] The teacher who expects a child to succeed probably creates a more intense relationship with the child, transmits the expectations, and facilitates success. Conversely, the teacher who expects a child to do poorly probably becomes part of the cause of the poor performance.

THE ORIENTAL PRECEDENT FOR THE EDUCATION MODEL

Students of Eastern cultures will have recognized that the educational model for human behavior is not original in any way. It has been part of Oriental cultures for many centuries. The inclusion of self-knowledge as part of educational curriculum is an essential part of both traditional and Zen Buddhism, of the Yoga system of Hinduism, and of some traditional Chinese philosophies. Eastern observers are fond of contrasting this learning, which they call wisdom, with the learning of Western education which they call simply knowledge. For these Eastern systems, a full understanding of the self, leading to self-acceptance, is the highest goal one can strive toward.

The concept of a tutor is also found in Eastern cultures. The Hindu seeks out a *guru* to teach him and the Buddhist apprentices himself to a monk. These men then teach you how to arrive at self-understanding. Several observers have already detailed those similarities with aspects of Western "psychotherapies";[36] the point here is simply to mention the fact that there is precedent in other cultures for synthesizing "psychotherapy" and traditional education within an educational model.

In summary, it would appear that the evidence for adding behavioral science to the curriculum and for using tutors (teachers chosen partly on the basis of their personality characteristics) is impressive. Its implications are that the important part of education (whether in school or in "therapy") is not *what* the teacher does, or how the teacher does it, but rather *who* the teacher is. Thus, it is not surprising to find that a thorough review of research on teaching methods failed to identify any method which could clearly be associated with either good or poor teaching.[37] The techniques of teaching, like the techniques of "therapy," are probably incidental to what takes place. Teachers and "therapists" should be selected primarily on the basis of their personality characteristics, not on their ability to pass organic chemistry or write a thesis. When this kind of selection begins, then "psychotherapy" and education will be fused; and students will learn to know themselves as well as they know other things.

10

Problems of Living Versus Brain Disease: "Schizophrenia" Revisited

WHAT kinds of people actually go to psychiatrists? Do they have brain diseases or do they, instead, have problems of living? The difference is more than a semantic sophism. Rather it has profound implications; for it determines what we do for these people, what they do for themselves, how we think of them, and how they think of themselves.

The first part of the book explored the disease model as it is currently applied to individuals claimed to be mentally "ill." In theoretical terms, this model was found to lead into a jungle of confusion. What happens when we move from theory to actually looking at individuals? Does a disease model help us understand their problems? Or is a problems-of-living model more appropriate?

The following are brief descriptions of twenty-eight people who typically end up in a psychiatrist's office. They are chosen to represent the whole range of problems which he sees.

PEOPLE WITH GENERAL PROBLEMS

   1. A young mother with two small children comes to a psychiatrist complaining that she is "depressed" and does not know "what life is worth living for." She married her husband, who is now a professional man, when she was only seventeen. She has vaguely contemplated suicide.

   2. A young woman whose husband is working overseas comes to a psychiatrist. She complains of strange

feelings—"like I am going crazy"—that are occurring increasingly often. On further questioning, it becomes clear that the feelings started shortly after her infant son was born.

3. A couple comes to a psychiatrist because of increasing problems in their marriage. She accuses him of being only interested in his academic career and other women. He accuses her of never reading a book and being frigid. They both agree that their marriage has gone progressively downhill over the past 2 years and that divorce is likely unless they can improve it.

4. A middle-aged man comes to a psychiatrist because of feelings of loneliness and sadness. He is a widower whose only child has recently moved away. He was also passed over 2 months ago for a promotion in his job and he is wondering if he is coming to the end of his productive career. He is considering suicide but only as a future possibility if things do not improve.

5. A middle-aged woman comes to a psychiatrist to get help with her habit of overeating. Several years previously she had been hypnotized and succeeded in losing 20 pounds in the following 2 months. She wants to know if it is possible to do that again. She does not complain of anything else.

6. A college student comes to a psychiatrist because of his inability to study. He had a brilliant academic background until the past year which was to have been his senior year. He is now on the verge of failing almost every course he is taking.

7. A young woman is encouraged to go to a psychiatrist by her mother following an abortion. Neither the mother nor the daughter has any real understanding of why the girl became pregnant when contraceptives were readily available. The mother has told her daughter that perhaps she wanted to.

8. A thirty-year-old woman comes to a psychiatrist because of her inability to get married. Each time she develops a relationship that starts to become serious,

she does something to destroy it. Most recently she picked up a hammer and threatened her boyfriend and he suggested that she seek psychiatric help.

9. An eight-year-old girl is brought to a psychiatrist by her mother. She has been increasingly aggressive toward her younger brother and started wetting her bed again since her father and mother recently separated. She has also complained of multiple stomach aches and headaches which the pediatrician says are "just emotional."

10. A twelve-year-old boy is referred to a psychiatrist by his school principal. He has become unmanageable in school and is doing failing work even though he is known to be intelligent. His mother brings him for the appointment very reluctantly.

These first ten vignettes represent the vast majority of people seen by psychiatrists. They are seen as "outpatients" by the psychiatrists in their private offices or clinics. Many psychiatrists, in fact, almost never see patients other than this group. According to the medical model, these people are "sick." They have "diseases." It is even possible for a psychiatrist to pick up his official "Diagnostic Classification of Mental Disorders" (lying under the stethoscope covered with dust) and produce a "disease" category for each of them. The list of "diseases" might look as follows:

1. Depressive neurosis
2. Anxiety neurosis
3. Marital maladjustment
4. Involutional melancholia or depressive neurosis
5. Psychophysiologic disorder
6. Specific learning disturbance with obsessive compulsive personality
7. Adjustment reaction of adolescence
8. Adjustment reaction of adult life with passive-aggressive personality
9. Adjustment reaction of childhood with psychophysiologic components
10. Hyperkinetic reaction of childhood

Of course, the selection of a proper "disease" is quite subjective; as was shown previously, another psychiatrist might choose a different list. Psychiatrists rarely worry about such things except when they must assign a "disease" to the patient so that the patient's insurance will pay the bill for the "medical" condition.

But does calling these people "sick" tell us anything useful about them? I think not. Rather it muddies the water irrevocably. Once people such as these are labeled as "sick," it becomes very difficult to help them in a logical manner since the "sickness" label carries with it a whole train of concomitant actions and reactions.

These people, rather than being "sick," have problems of living. Other words which convey their predicaments are words like crises, social disturbances, interpersonal or intrapersonal problems, and adjustment problems. They do not have pain but rather unhappiness. They do not have problems with their anatomy but rather problems with their thoughts, feelings, and behavior. They have the same problems that all of us have—maybe more, maybe less. To call them "sick" implies that they are in a different category of persons than ourselves who are "well." We know these people and we know that they are not different. We are those people. And if they are "sick," then the "sickroll" corresponds exactly to the census roll.

Since these people are not "sick," they do not need to be "cured." They *do* need to learn more about their problems of living, however. They do not need a doctor to learn from, but rather a tutor—a warm, empathetic individual who has been selected partly on the basis of personality characteristics and life experience and has been trained broadly in the behavioral sciences. The tutor would also have been trained to recognize signs of organic brain disease in order to be able to recognize the rare cases of medical conditions (e.g., brain tumors) which present problems of living; such training can be done in a few weeks. By meeting with a tutor, such people could learn why they are thinking, feeling, and doing the things that they define as a problem. Through such understanding, they could learn how to modify their thoughts, feelings, and actions.

PEOPLE WHO HAVE SEXUAL PROBLEMS

11. A young man comes to a psychiatrist wanting to know if anything can be done about his homosexuality. The man has had homosexual relationships since he was 15; his only attempt at a heterosexual relationship, he found disgusting. He has a good job and is finishing work on a master's degree.

12. A middle-aged man is sent to a psychiatrist by his attorney. The man has been arrested for peeping in windows at night. This is the man's second arrest. The attorney thought it would look better in court if his client was seeking psychiatric help. The man has little interest in learning why he feels compelled to peep.

These two men represent a large group of people whose sexual practices have been labeled as "deviant" by our society. Only a few of them ever encounter a psychiatrist and fewer still change their behavior as a result of such an encounter. They are labeled as "sick" both by society in general and by psychiatrists in particular. The official "Diagnostic Classification of Mental Disorders" currently lists nine different varieties of sexual "deviations," to wit: "homosexuality,"* "fetishism," "pedophilia," "transvestitism," "exhibitionism," "voyeurism," "sadism," "masochism," and "other." It does not specify whether "heterosexuality" might be included as a "disease" under "other."

In terms of numbers, it is estimated that there are 4 million men in the United States who are exclusively homosexual and another 6 million who engage in sexual activity with both sexes regularly. Without even adding the "lesbians," "exhibitionists," and others, it is apparent that this is a "disease" of epidemic proportions.

Homosexuality and the other sexual "deviations" are, of course, not real diseases at all. They are ways that people choose to relate to other people sexually. As such, they are merely part of a spectrum of choices open to us. Some are common choices, some uncommon choices, but none are diseases.

*In December 1973, the Board of Trustees of the American Psychiatric Association finally voted to remove "homosexuality" from the list of mental "diseases."

To say that people "choose" a certain form of sexual expression does not necessarily imply a conscious element in operation. Our choices of the way we will relate sexually are usually a product of many things, some of which may be biological and many of which are clearly related to our early experience. Thus a boy may "choose" to relate to men rather than women sexually because the woman he knows best, his mother, is a shrew, or because his body chemistry inclines him to be more attracted to men.

If sexual "deviations" like homosexuality are not diseases, then what are they? They are simply behavior, part of the behavior associated with relating to others. They usually are not even problems of living except under two circumstances:

1. If the person himself feels guilty: In this case, he may have a problem of living which he needs help with. The help may consist of either relieving the guilt or changing the behavior so that he will not feel guilty. The young man above represents this problem of living, for it was his guilt which took him to the psychiatrist.

2. If his behavior is harmful to others: Examples of this might be the man above who is peeping in windows, a man who exhibits himself to small girls, or a homosexual who solicits partners among young boys. In these instances, the person certainly does have a problem because society prohibits such activity. He needs help with his problem. And if he cannot control his behavior, then he should be dealt with by the legal system as will be described later. But in no case does calling him "sick" add anything except a pejorative label and the illusory reassurance that he certainly is not like us since we are "well."

Furthermore, since we dropped our puritanical veils, we have become more aware of the wide range of behavior that may occur under the title of "heterosexual." We know that many people have difficulty achieving mutually satisfactory heterosexual relationships and that hiding beneath the bed are a whole panoply of premature ejaculations, degrees of frigidity, and varieties of sexual selfishness. These people too have problems of living for which they need help. Looked at broadly, then, it is not the person's *choice* of sexual expression which determines whether or not he has problems, but rather his ability to achieve a satisfactory relationship within that choice.

PEOPLE WHO WANT TO COMMIT SUICIDE

13. A young woman is brought to a psychiatrist by police who were called by her mother. The girl took five sleeping pills, then called her boyfriend, and said she had just taken them. The boyfriend called her mother, who in turn called the police. The girl now admits that she doesn't really want to die.

14. A forty-year-old divorcee is admitted to the hospital in a coma, following a suicide attempt with large amounts of sleeping pills. Three days later, after she has recovered, a psychiatrist is asked to see her. It is clear that she expected to die and it was only a chance visit by her landlord that resulted in her being found before she was dead. She insists now that she still wants to die.

These two women are both suicidal although in quite different ways. The teenaged girl is using the threat of suicide to manipulate people and to call attention to the fact that she needs help. Her gesture is a cry for help. She is not "sick" in any sense of the word. Rather she is choosing one method of calling attention to her predicament. If she does not get help, she may, at a later date, reach the stage of being seriously suicidal.

The second woman has reached that latter stage. She has clearly decided that she wants to die. Women like her are seen far less frequently by a psychiatrist. For every person who has made a serious suicide attempt, psychiatrists see four or five who are not really trying to kill themselves but rather are crying for help.

Should this second woman be called "sick"? Since she wants to die, this is the label we pin on her in our culture. It gives us the right not only to stop her, but to put her in a "hospital" and keep her there *indefinitely* until she either changes her mind or *tells us* that she has changed her mind. That is the present situation—a seriously suicidal person can be kept in a "hospital" for as long as she continues to tell the "doctor" that she wants to die. In many states, this can legally be forever. Of course it never is; for the seriously suicidal person learns the rules of the game quickly and tells her "doctor" what a mistake she has made and how much she wants to live. She is then discharged and goes out and commits suicide. The whole series of events often takes on a ritual appearance, a pantomime on the shore of the river Styx with the psychiatrist playing the role of Harlequin.

If this woman is "sick," then she has a very common "disease"; for about 24,000 people commit suicide each year in the United States alone.[2] Calling such people "sick" solves some complex problems that we would rather not face. If this woman is "sick," then her action is presumably not rational. We do not have to address the terrible implications of her act. If she is not "sick," what does her act say about the quality of our lives? What does it say about the abyss between our illusory happiness and our reality of despair? What does it say about the human condition? Yes—it is certainly safer to call such people "sick." Then whatever it is that they have perceived, we do not have to pay attention to in ourselves.

We know now, of course, that this woman has chosen only one way to commit suicide. She is doing it openly and calling it by its proper name. It is this open confrontation that we will not countenance. Embedded as we are in our Judeo-Christian tradition, we insist that a person who tells us that they want to die must be "sick." There are many other forms of suicide that we do accept however—as long as the person disguises it and does not confront us openly. Drug experimentation may often be an attempt at suicide ("No, I don't know what kind of pills I took. No, I didn't really care much one way or the other whether I woke up.") Drug addiction certainly is a form of suicide—the unfeeling, twilight state of a person "high" on heroin is very close to death. And many of the "accidental overdosages" are anything but accidental. Excessive overeating and alcoholism can be forms of suicide, as can be deliberate overworking. People who are "accident prone" are usually suicidal—witness the "freeway freaks" who pass you every day. People who neglect their body may also want to die; for example, the diabetic who keeps "forgetting" his insulin and going into a coma. Suicide must also be looked for in war, both among the volunteers for the dangerous missions and the Dr. Strangeloves who sit behind the lines and escalate things. When suicide is thus put in its true perspective, the line between who is "sick" and who is "well" becomes blurred indeed.[3] In fact, the concept of "sick" loses meaning altogether.

PEOPLE WHO LOSE THEIR MEMORY

15. A young man walks into the emergency room of a hospital and asks to see a psychiatrist. He says he cannot remember who he is or how he got to the hospital. He only remembers "waking up" on the lawn outside the hospital. He has no identification on him. An internist examines him and can find no signs of injury or illness.

This young man represents a kind of problem that psychiatrists see infrequently. He has completely lost his memory. Other people may have only partial memory loss and still others forget only the time around a specific event. To call the man "sick" and label him as "acute hysterical neurosis, dissociative type" does nothing at all for our understanding. Rather, it acts as an epithet which obstructs understanding by promoting the illusion that the man has a "disease."

Although the young man is not "sick," he does have many problems of living. He has a wife and a child that he does not really want. He has borrowed money that he cannot repay. He has had a recent homosexual experience that has made him worry that he might be a homosexual. And he does not know what kind of work he wants to do or what he wants out of life. These are indeed problems—problems of living. And he needs immediate and abundant help with them. But this is a far cry from saying that he has a "disease."

The closing off of his mind is an unconscious solution to all these problems. He did not decide consciously to do it—it just happened. He might have tried other solutions—suicide was one that he had contemplated. So his state of complete loss of memory is an attempted solution to his problems. Since it is not an especially effective or efficient solution, the role of the tutor who helps him would be to work toward alternative solutions.

PEOPLE WHO ARE ADDICTED

16. A man in his early thirties is sent to a psychiatrist by his wife. He has had increasing problems because of his drinking, most recently resulting in a car accident and the loss of his job. Two brief hospital admissions for delirium tremens, one of the medical complications of alcoholism, has not slowed him down at all.
17. A twenty-year-old man is sent to a psychiatrist by his social worker. He has been addicted to heroin for 2 years and says he wants to break the addiction. To support his habit, he has managed a ring of teenaged boys who stole $200 worth of goods a day from stores.

These two men represent a large group of people who are addicted. They see psychiatrists but usually because they are forced to. Only occasionally do addicts seek out psychiatrists on their own. Their numbers are large. In the United States, there are estimated to be 6 million alcohol addicts and ½ million heroin addicts.

Addictions can take many forms, from gambling and overeating to alcohol and heroin. Common to them all are the compulsive nature of the behavior and the self-destructive aspect of it. The addict will go on and on even when it becomes clear that his behavior is destroying him. Freud believed that even masturbation was an addiction; in fact, he called it the "primal addiction" and said that addiction to cigarettes, alcohol, and drugs were merely substitutes for masturbation.[4] This was, of course, during the enlightened period of psychiatric history when masturbation was thought to cause insanity.

Not only are people who are addicted accepted as "diseased" but this acceptance is growing. MacAndrews, in his essay "On the Notion That Certain Persons Who Are Given To Frequent Drunkenness Suffer from a Disease Called Alcoholism," concludes that: "One is an alcoholic by virtue of the fact that a *bona fide* member of the medical profession, acting in his capacity as a member of that profession, has so designated him."[5] In other words, an alcoholic becomes an alcoholic when a doctor calls him one; up until then he is merely an individual who has a problem of drinking too much.

The legal implications of accepting addiction as a disease are profound and can only be touched upon here. Following logically from the disease model, a court recently declared that drug addicts, because they are "sick," cannot be punished for their addiction. "Narcotics addiction is a form of insanity, rendering the subject incapable of committing the offense alleged, so that it is denial of due process and equal protection of the laws to punish him for the offense."[6] Logically, then, the drug addict cannot be punished for stealing to obtain money for drugs (thus making three-quarters of the thefts in New York City not prosecutable) and the alcoholic cannot be punished for drunken driving. It is little wonder that there has been some resistance to efforts by psychiatrists and well-meaning legislators to have alcohol and drug abusers clearly and permanently labeled as "diseased." The average citizen recognizes the absurdity of this and can no more accept it than he could accept masturbation being labeled as an addiction and "disease." Perhaps that will be proposed next.

The "disease" concept of addiction leads down a path both absurd and chaotic. One implication is that "treatment" may be made mandatory. There is no evidence that *forced* "treatment" of either condition makes the slightest difference in the long run. Addicts who *want* guidance, on the other hand, can get assistance from people who will help them solve their problems of living—people like tutors.

Moreover, calling addicts "sick" is a method of disguising the more important question of *why* a person becomes an addict. Granted, he has a craving for the drug (a physiological addiction); that is simply a phenomenon related to the addiction but it is no explanation. Why should 6 million Americans prefer the daily drunken stupor of alcohol to reality? Why should many residents in ghetto areas of our cities prefer to live in the twilight of a heroin "high"? Are all these people "sick"? If so, then we can disregard their action and send them somewhere to get "treatment." If they are not "sick," then they are like us. And their problems are our problems.

The medical model of addiction may also act, paradoxically, to reinforce addiction. Insofar as addicts are "sick" and have a "disease" of the brain, then they are not themselves responsible. Their addiction is caused by mysterious chemical forces that have taken control and they are the helpless victims of their "disease." This is the reason that most addicts, both on alcohol and narcotics, will quickly agree with the medical model. The alternative model implies that they are responsible for their addiction and that they have chosen it as their means for dealing with the problems of living. For an addict, it is the difference between being able to project the cause of his behavior into a "disease" scapegoat or having to accept the responsibility himself.

Finally, the medical model reinforces the need of many addicts to degrade themselves. The self-destructive aspect of addiction, partly as a form of "hidden suicide," has been mentioned previously. The medical model saddles the addict with a "disease," thereby putting him in the same category as someone who has cancer or leprosy. This is very comfortable for most addicts, for it is part of their self-image. To deprive them of their "disease" and tell them that they simply have problems of living like everybody else (but which they are handling in a particular way) would be to offer them dignity that is contrary to their self-image. In summary, then, not only is the medical model illogical for people who are addicted, but it probably reinforces their addiction as well. These people need help, but they do not need doctors.

PEOPLE WITH LOW INTELLIGENCE

18. A teen-aged boy is brought to a psychiatrist by his parents. He has been previously diagnosed as "mentally retarded" and has been living at home. Recently, however, he has been setting small fires in the neighborhood and the neighbors have complained that he is becoming a nuisance.

This boy represents another large group of people in our society who are seen by a psychiatrist. He is seen just once, however—to be "evaluated" and then assigned to an institution to spend the rest of his life.

The boy is "mentally retarded." That means that he was born (or became) less intelligent than the majority of people. Sometimes the lower intelligence is based upon an early injury or disease; in the majority of cases, however, it is associated with social and environmental deprivation. There are over 6 million people so labeled in the United States and, at any one time, 215,000 of them are confined to institutions.

"Mental retardation" is officially classified as a "disease" under the ultimate authority of psychiatrists. Unofficially, however, greater headway has been made in moving beyond the "disease" concept for this condition than for many others. Increasingly frequently, this group of people are being referred to as simply part of the continuum of intelligence, not as a separate group. This is promising insofar as it has gone. It is just as logical to cut off the top 10 percent of the intelligence spectrum and say that the group has the "disease" of "mental progression" as it is to cut off the bottom 10 percent and call it "mental retardation."

This is not to say that people with very low intelligence do not have problems. Depending upon how low their intelligence is, they may have severe problems. Some are even unable to provide food and shelter for themselves. These are very real and practical problems. Another set of problems, of course, arises out of the fact that they are labeled as "mentally retarded." The consequences of wearing this badge are devastating. These problems of living do not constitute "sickness," however.

There is also no question that many people with low intelligence need a place where they can go periodically, or even to live for long periods, which does not make the demands upon them that modern technological society does. They are just one of several groups of people who need this. Such a place— a retreat—should be available to anyone on a voluntary basis. It should be an educational institution to obviate and assist with problems of living. More will be said about retreats in the following chapter. Here it is only necessary to note that institutions for the "mentally retarded" are often called "schools" or "training schools." Thus, except for their involuntary and custodial character they are a little closer to the idea of a retreat than state "hospitals" are.

PEOPLE WHO HAVE BECOME OLD

19. A seventy-five-year-old man is brought to a psychiatrist by the police because he has been found wandering in the street and cannot remember where he lives. This is the third time that the police have found him this week. The man apparently has no family.

This man has grown old. As part of the process of aging, he has had changes in the arteries carrying the blood supply to his brain. The blood supply is no longer as good as it once was. Consequently, certain functions of the brain, like memory, are impaired.

To say the man is "sick" is inaccurate. There is no disease process per se. Rather, the changes are part of the aging process, natural developments that are found in all people as they age. Some people show it more than others—some people start to have a failing memory at sixty and in others it may not begin until they are eighty-five.

We have done these people a grave disservice in our society by labeling them as "sick." The official designation is "nonpsychotic organic brain syndrome with senile or presenile brain disease" or "nonpsychotic organic brain syndrome with circulatory disturbance." Translated into English this means that the person is old. But by so labeling them, we put them into the category of "sick" people and acquire the right to "hospitalize" them.

The "hospitalization" of people who have grown old is a parody on words, but a cruel one. Since there is no possibility of "treatment" for such people (i.e., they are not going to regain their memory), the use of a "hospital" is, by definition, a hoax. Of all the people who we presently are labeling as mentally "ill" and thereby assigning to "hospitals," no group has been more dishonored than those who have grown old. There are over one-half million such people in "nursing homes" and another 150,000 in state "hospitals." The fact that many of them die shortly after they are sent to these places is the only logical response—they take one look at their "hospital" and decide that it is better to be dead!

People who have grown old are not "sick," but they certainly do have problems. They have problems of getting food and shelter, problems remembering whether they turned off the stove, and problems remembering where they live. Many of them also have problems because they are lonely or neglected or no longer appreciated for their skills. These problems cannot be solved by pasting "sick" labels on the people and trundling them off to "hospitals." On the other hand, the problems might be alleviated if, in addition to social services and appropriate housing, tutors were available to help these people learn how to live with their failing memories and decreasing abilities.

PEOPLE OUTSIDE THE MAINSTREAM

20. A middle-aged man is sent to a psychiatrist by an internist. The man has multiple symptoms, mostly relating to fears about his heart; but the internist thinks it is all "in his head." The man has been in and out of the Veterans Administration Hospital for 10 years. Each time he leaves, he gets progressively more frightened and is readmitted 2 or 3 months later. He has no family and no job skills. In the hospital, he is happy and helps in the kitchen.

21. An elderly man is brought in to see a psychiatrist by the police. He has been picked up for vagrancy with no money, family, or place to stay. He admits to having been in and out of Veterans Administration Hospitals from Maine to California and in fact appears to make a seasonal round of them.

These two men represent a very large group of people whom psychiatrists see briefly, usually just long enough to sign their readmission papers to a "hospital" of one kind or another. They are the people who are out of the mainstream of our society—the people drifting along in the side eddies both unnoticed and unnoticing. For them, the miracle of their birth is a heavy yoke to be dragged from day to day. The milestones of growth, family, and holidays with which the majority of us mark our lives are but pebbles to them or dim memories that were aborted in some distant past.

We presently call these people "sick" and have a whole array of labels for them from which we can choose. The most popular are "schizoid personality" and "inadequate personality." The "sickness" category then allows us to put them into "hospitals." Contrary to most of the other "sick" groups we have been discussing, however, these people often *seek* admission to "hospitals." The Veterans Administration "hospitals" are full of them. They produce many of the paradoxes of mental "hospitals" that were described in Chapter 5 with "patients" trying to stay in for as long as they can—strange "hospitals" indeed!

The number of such people is unknown but is certainly in the millions. They are the constant core of the deserted inner city, the steady clientele of the Salvation Army, and the backbone of our prisons. In the last, they are the prisoners who are in for the pettiest crimes but who seem to enjoy it; they have even been known to go out and commit a small robbery in October so that they will have a warm home for the winter. They also are abundant in our mental "hospitals." It is estimated that up to one-quarter of mental "hospital" beds are occupied by them.

To call such people "sick" is absurdness *in extremis*. It is like calling a ladder "sick" for being too short to reach the roof. It is like calling a bicycle "sick" for being unable to go 100 miles an hour. Our use of the adjective "sick" for such people shows only our own arrogance in believing that the mainstream as we define it is "well." The increasing numbers of younger people dropping out of society's mainstream should give us pause to reconsider whether we are right.

Many of these people do have problems that they need help with. Others have none and ask only to be left alone. For those who need help with their problems, it should be available. And there should be places where they can go and live if they want to—not "hospitals" but retreats.

PEOPLE WITH BRAIN DISEASE

Up to this point, we have been describing the people for whom the medical model is clearly not appropriate and who have been mislabeled. We now turn to the small percentage of mentally "ill" people at the other end of the spectrum for whom the medical model is accurate. These few people really are sick. Two examples follow:

22. A middle-aged man is sent by an internist to a psychiatrist for an opinion on his mental condition. The internist suspects that the man has the late effects of syphilis of the brain. Prior to seeing the internist, the man had become increasingly forgetful and at times believed that his wife was trying to poison him. The psychiatrist confirms the diagnosis of syphilis and returns the man to the internist for treatment.

23. An elderly woman is urged to go to a psychiatrist by her daughter because of increasingly bizarre behavior. In the previous week, for instance, this very proper woman had approached two men on the street and propositioned them. The psychiatrist suspects a brain disease of some kind and sends the woman to a neurologist who diagnoses a brain tumor.

These two people both have brain diseases. One has syphilis and the other has a brain tumor. The disease process in these brains has produced changes which are affecting behavior and thinking. No doubt the people have problems of living too, but such problems are distinctly secondary to the disease. Because they have true brain diseases, they need the care of doctors.

This is the part of mental "illness" which really does belong in the medical model. It is not a large part, however. At the most, brain diseases like syphilis and tumors constitute 5 percent of people occupying beds in mental "hospitals." For a psychiatrist seeing patients in private practice, the percentage would be much lower.

It is often said that because this group exists—that is, because a small percentage of people labeled as mentally "ill" actually do have brain diseases—then a doctor must care for all people with similar behavior. In other words, because this group with true brain diseases may have symptoms like the other group, who do not have brain diseases, then a doctor must be in charge of both in order to decide which is which. This is simply not true. As mentioned previously, it is possible to train a tutor or anyone with a behavioral science background to be able to detect probable true brain disease. There are a series of signs and symptoms which a person can be taught to look for. Such training can be done in only a few weeks and could be part of a behavioral science training course. Then if a question arose while a tutor was assessing a person with an apparent problem of living, a doctor could be called in to confirm or deny the diagnosis of brain disease.

"SCHIZOPHRENIA REVISITED"

In looking at people who see a psychiatrist, we have tried to assess whether a medical model or an educational model best describes them. Up to this point, we have found that at least 75 percent of people previously called mentally "ill" do not warrant that label and that a maximum of 5 percent do. The former group includes at least 4 million people who are homosexual, 6 million people with low intelligence, 6 million people addicted to alcohol, one-half million people addicted to heroin, up to one million people who have grown old, an unknown number of people outside the mainstream of society, and several thousand people who want to commit suicide. This is a lot of mislabeling and it is rapidly expanding. It has been called the "kingdom of therapy.'"

What does this leave of mental "illness"? It leaves a remaining 20 percent of people that we label as mentally "ill" because they have problems with reality. In medical language, they are referred to as "psychotics." Some examples follow:

24. A young woman is brought to a psychiatrist by the police. Her husband has observed her watching the neighbor's house for hours at a time with binoculars. Furthermore, she has talked increasingly frequently about a plot against her by Communists whom she suspects of living in that house.

25. A teen-aged boy is brought to a psychiatrist by his father. The boy has withdrawn from the family and spends days in his room alone. When spoken to he often appears not to hear. Recently he has been observed speaking to someone in his room although there is nobody there.

26. A successful businessman is brought to a psychiatrist by his wife because "he's become very high." Within the previous month, he has bought and sold three businesses, all at considerable loss, and is now negotiating to sell out altogether to a rival corporation. Simultaneously, he has purchased two new cars, a washer and dryer, and a summer cabin, none of which his family needed.

27. A forty-year-old woman is brought to a psychiatrist by her husband. She has been cared for at home by him for several years, although when she was younger she spent 10 years in a mental "hospital." Recently she has been staying in bed all the time, refusing to eat, and urinating in the corner of her room.

28. A middle-aged man is brought to a psychiatrist by his mother. He has been in and out of mental "hospitals" since he was twenty-two. At home, he has recently started refusing to take his medicine or to do his chores around the farm. He is almost completely unable to think of things as abstracts but rather sees them concretely.

These five people represent the remainder of those whom we label mentally "ill." They constitute 20 percent of first admissions to mental "hospitals" and many stay on to spend most of their lives in these institutions. For most psychiatrists in private practice, this group comprises much less than 20 percent of their practice.[8]

The official labels put on these people are variations of the category "psychosis." For the five people described above, the most likely labels would be "paranoid schizophrenia," "simple schizophrenia," "manic-depressive psychosis," and for the last two "residual schizophrenia." These labels are impressive and convey to the uninitiated the idea that we know what we are talking about.

Unfortunately, this is not the case. We still do not know whether "schizophrenia" is a single brain disease or several brain diseases with a final common pathway. What appears to be increasingly clear, however, is that classical "schizophrenia" *is* indeed a brain disease and not caused by a cold, rejecting mother; an unresolved oedipus complex; or ambiguous messages from the parent to the child. By "classical schizophrenics" I mean those whom virtually everyone can agree upon—those whose illness begins insidiously in early adulthood, with flat emotions, delusions and/or hallucinations, and intermittent stays in the hospital throughout their lives.

The evidence that these people have a true brain disease has become increasingly strong in recent years. In one study, 60 percent of "schizophrenics" were shown to have neurological impairment, a sign that some disease process or damage was occurring in their central nervous system.[9] Other studies have emphasized the frequent appearance of "schizophrenia-like" symptoms in people who have known physical diseases affecting their brains.[10] Many "schizophrenics" have been shown to have abnormal proteins in their blood and spinal fluid,[11] or altered enzymes like creatine phosphokinase and aldolase.[12] The author's personal research has been on the possibility of a virus as the primary causative agent of "schizophrenia," which would explain such phenomena as the "schizophrenics" who develop a high fever and suddenly die (called fatal catatonia) and the fact that there is a seasonally higher incidence of schizophrenic births in the first 3 months of the year.[13]

Moreover, the expanding field of orthomolecular psychiatry is also based upon the premise that "schizophrenia" is an organic brain disease. Supporters of this school stress the fact that slight changes in the molecular concentration of common substances in the brain may, in a genetically predisposed person, cause changes in the person's perception of his environment.[14] This "metabolic dysperception" then leads to secondary changes, including disorders of thinking and behavior which are characteristic of "schizophrenics." Although psychiatrists following the orthomolecular approach prescribe large doses of vitamins and strict diet control in addition to more traditional drugs for the cure of the disease, these therapeutic adjuncts have not been shown to be superior in controlled studies except in a small subgroup of "schizophrenics." Further studies are in progress to clarify this. The most important contribution of orthomolecular psychiatry may turn out not to be its emphasis on megavitamin therapy, but rather its stress on "schizophrenia" as an organic brain disease and on altered perception by the brain as the primary brain defect in the development of the disease. The altered perception could be caused by one or several different causative agents.

A conviction that "schizophrenia" is an organic brain disease unites all research referred to above. In addition, other research has pointed toward an organic (at least genetic) causation for some cases of "manic-depressive psychosis."[15] As continuing research clarifies the organic aspects of some "psychoses," then those which are truly brain diseases will be turned over to the neurologists for treatment. They won't be called "schizophrenics" or "manic depressives" anymore, of course, since the real cause of the illness(es) will be known and so named. Since neurologists are specialists in diseases of the brain and since neurology is a true medical speciality, this is entirely appropriate. Many present-day psychiatrists will probably elect to remain in medicine as neurologists and work with this group of patients. Other psychiatrists, who enjoy teaching people about problems of living more than treating brain diseases, will elect to become behavioral scientists.

All of this sounds straightforward enough to do, and would be, if only we had the definitive research answers on causes of "schizophrenia" as a brain disease. Unfortunately we do not. Moreover the scene becomes further confused by the fact that many individuals can be forced into a temporary reactive "psychosis" if subjected to overwhelming stress. Such individuals are seen under conditions of war and disaster, among immigrants, among Peace Corps Volunteers, or among anyone who must accommodate to massive sudden changes in their lives. Such individuals may appear to be "schizophrenic" for brief periods, but rapidly return to normal when removed from the stress. They should not be thought of as having a primary brain disease but rather as being overwhelmed by their acute problems of living.

Another element which further muddles the scene is the way in which the term "schizophrenia" has come to be used, especially in the United States and the Soviet Union. Some professionals will label as "schizophrenic" virtually anyone who looks cross-eyed or wears different colored socks. Labels like "borderline schizophrenic," "latent schizophrenic," or "pseudoneurotic schizophrenic" are used. As such the term has become almost meaningless and its demise, along with that of psychiatry itself, will be a welcome addition to clarity of thought. Those "schizophrenics" who have true brain disease will be so labeled and treated. And those "schizophrenics" who don't have a brain disease but rather have severe problems of living will also be so labeled and offered help with their problems wherever possible. The term "schizophrenia" will wither away to the shelves of museums, looked back upon as an historical curiosity along with the crank telephone.

None of this means that people with true "schizophrenia" and other forms of brain disease do not have problems of living as well. Nor does it mean that people with overwhelming problems of living may not benefit from the occasional use of medication. What it does mean is that we must be clear about what the primary difficulty is—disease or problems—and offer the person appropriate help. The paranoid woman described above has alienated all her friends because of her suspiciousness and so has nobody to talk to. The withdrawn teen-aged boy is being pressured by his parents to go on to college because they think that will help him. The businessman who has been "high" is on the verge of financial disaster. And the older woman and man are not able to provide for their own needs.

These are serious problems of living which are the result of, not the cause of, the brain disease. As such, they are similar to problems of living concomitant to other medical diseases. Examples of this are the problems that a child diabetic may have because of severe restrictions in food or activity, or the problems of blindness for a person who has eye disease.

To begin to differentiate medical problems from human problems in this manner is long overdue. The present scene finds many doctors, trained in medicine, spending the majority of their time "treating" problems of living. This is not only wasteful of medical talents but produces appropriate help for human problems on only a random basis. To say that all doctors should also be tutors and do both jobs is socially and economically inefficient; it would be like advocating that doctors should teach blind people how to read braille just because the doctors also treat their eye diseases. "Psychotics" should have their brain disease treated by a doctor in the same way as a diabetic or ulcer patient is treated by a doctor, but the problems of living in all three cases can be better helped by a tutor, selected on the basis of personality characteristics and life experience and trained in the behavioral sciences.

While it is readily acknowledged that we do not yet have the expertise to make precise distinctions between truly brain-diseased "schizophrenics" and the others who have no brain disease, it is important that we make a beginning in this direction. And until we have more precise indicators, it is best that we err on the side of labeling too few, rather than too many, as brain diseased. In other words, a person should be assumed *not* to have a brain disease until proven otherwise on the basis of probability. This is exactly the opposite of what we do now as we blithely label everyone who behaves a little oddly as "schizophrenic." Human dignity rather demands that people be assumed to be in control of their behavior and not brain diseased unless there is strong evidence to the contrary.

In an historical sense, one should be aware of the irony of all this. During a period of time when the medical model of human behavior was supreme, the predominant theories of causation for "schizophrenia" were based on intrapersonal and interpersonal conflict—in other words, not on medical theories at all. And now, with the advocating of the death of psychiatry and thus the medical model of human behavior, we return to medical theories to explain some cases of "schizophrenia." Ironic it is; but if it leads to a more coherent and effective solution to these medical and human problems, it will also be more useful.

NORMALITY REVISED

The problem of normality discussed in Chapter 4 ceases to be a problem as soon as the medical model is put to rest. People with problems of living become part of a continuum with everyone since everyone has such problems. Some may have bigger problems, or different kinds of problems, but there is no implied segregation into those who are not diseased (= normal) and those who are diseased (= abnormal). Thus under an educational model, arguments about normality would become superfluous.

Of course, certain kinds of behavior will always be found more commonly than others. It is probable, for instance, that a person whose major sexual satisfaction comes from dressing up in clothing of the opposite sex will always be looked upon as different, since this behavior occurs very infrequently. It could be said that this person's behavior is unusual in the sense that it occurs statistically infrequently, but this is not to say that it is "abnormal." Such behavior may be said to be odd, strange, or eccentric but it could not be called "abnormal" in anything other than a statistical sense. This would allow for the natural diversity among human beings whose limited functioning in some areas of their lives may be combined with more than average functioning in other areas. An example is Van Gogh who was periodically limited in his ability to perceive reality but who was extraordinarily richly endowed with artistic creativity.

Of course, any given behavior may be declared illegal by a society if it does not want to condone that particular behavior. For instance, a society could make it illegal to dress up in clothing of the opposite sex just as many parts of our society have declared homosexual relations to be illegal. A society has the right to do this if the majority of its members so desire. But it should be done judicially—declaring the behavior illegal—and not rationalized medically by declaring the behavior to be "sick."

Dropping normality as a behavioral concept also removes, once and for all, the artificial categories to which we consign behavior that differs from ours. We all become part of the same world, each with peculiarities or aberrations of behavior but each related to one another. Either we are *all* normal, in this sense, or "...we are left with a being like ourselves, a half-crazed creature more or less adjusted to a mad world. This is normality in our present age."[16]

11

Clients, Retreats, and the Educational Contract

How can a neo-educational model, complete with behavioral science and tutors, be applied to the large numbers of people who have problems of living? What practical problems can be anticipated?

The first thing that is needed is a suitable name for the people with problems of living. Names are important, for they carry both implications and connotations. Therefore, the word "patients" must be discarded, for it implies that people with problems of living are in some way "sick." One possibility is simply to call them people with problems of living. Another is to call them clients or students. The term "client," used by Carl Rogers and others, connotes a private contractual relationship to help solve a specific problem. A good example of the use of client in this way is in the legal profession. The term "student" is more appropriate in the context of an educational institution. Both could be used to convey the sense of a person who has a problem of living and wants to learn more about it.

Places are also needed in which the self-education of students and clients can take place. As long as they are in school, in an ideal world, the self-education would be occurring there in a series of behavioral science courses or seminars. By the time students finished formal schooling, they would know as much about human behavior as about any other area of study. They would know as much about why people are aggressive as they do about how to find the area of a triangle, as much about mechanisms people use to increase self-esteem as about the capital city of each state. They would have an understanding of the antecedents of human behavior, both those arising in intrapsychic processes as well as those coming from social and cultural forces. The study of human behavior in the schools would have a separate identity as a legitimate subject for study. The alternative, to have it pervade all courses, suffers from the shortcoming that anything which is supposed to pervade everything in school quickly becomes so thin it evaporates.

RETREATS

Once formal schooling is finished, then education on problems of living could occur anywhere. A client could seek out a tutor, arrange the educational contract with him, and proceed. For many people, however, there would be a need for an additional institution after formal schooling was finished. Such an institution could be called a retreat.

Retreats would be completely voluntary institutions which might be available in a variety of forms and sizes. Common to them all would be their voluntary nature; there would be no such thing as having been "sent" to a retreat. Another characteristic would be the self-governing nature of them. The people who live there, both short-term and long-term, would set up and administer their own rules. There would be no doctor or behavioral scientist in charge. The degree of shared living facilities would probably vary widely from retreat to retreat and even within the same retreat.

Connected with each retreat would be a series of sheltered workshops and opportunities to learn job skills. Also available would be courses on human behavior and problems of living. Depending upon the number of behavioral scientists available, there would be more or less individual tutoring on problems of living. Strong emphasis, however, would be put upon each individual's ability and obligation to help other people in the retreat. Thus, much of the education that would occur at a retreat would be among the people who chose to live there.

The people there would probably include a wide variety. They would all share one need, however—the need to get away from the mechanized, competitive, and rapidly moving life in the mainstream. They might wish to use the retreat for only a few days or they might want to stay for a few years. Since there would no longer be any mental "hospitals," it is probable that retreats would be attractive alternatives for many of the people presently inhabiting such institutions. Thus there would be a combination of people who have grown old, people with low intelligence, people who are addicted to alcohol or narcotics, and people outside the mainstream generally. Added to these would be others who need to escape for a short or long period of time from society, people who need an opportunity to resolve personal crises, and people who just want to stop long enough to figure out what life is all about.

The need for retreats has been clearly and poignantly shown as some state mental "hospitals" have closed. The people who have been in these "hospitals" have often been released to the communities without any alternative facilities being provided. The result is that they end up in third-class boarding houses or hotels unable to care for themselves. It is estimated that 12,000 former mental "patients" inhabit the Bowery area of New York City, living by making the rounds of soup kitchens and the Salvation Army.[1] And not coincidentally, the City of New York concluded that what was needed was a "retreat" which they set up in the Catskill Mountains north of the city.[2] It has facilities for a thousand people and over half of these remain there more-or-less permanently. It is completely voluntary.

Trying to force individuals of low intelligence out of the state institutions and into the community, although often done with the best of intentions, has also shown the need for retreats. Such individuals are often cheated, robbed, and otherwise victimized when they try and live alone in large cities.[3] Ideally they should have alternate, voluntary facilities available to them where they can be safe, where counseling regarding the problems of living would be available, and from which they can freely come and go.

The idea of retreats is certainly not new. Even traditional mental "hospitals" sometimes incorporate the concept although in name only, e.g., the Brattleboro Retreat, the Institute for Living. Many of the new ideas inherent in "therapeutic communities" in mental "hospitals" are a step in this direction; although as long as the community is "therapeutic," it is by definition constricted by the medical model.[4] The idea of a retreat is also developed by Braginsky, Braginsky, and Ring in *Methods of Madness: The Mental Hospital as a Last Resort.* They describe the need for a retreat as a place where people can go for renewal "without having to use the currency of self-respect and self-esteem" by having to define themselves as "patients."[5]

On the practical side, the buildings which would be used as retreats would be provided by the local, state, or federal government. It would be accepted that this was a governmental responsibility—to provide its citizens with a place where they can, literally, retreat. Since the opening of retreats would coincide with the closing of all mental "hospitals," it seems reasonable to assume that the same buildings or campuses might be used in many instances, at least initially. Though this would make the distinction between "hospitals" and retreats more difficult for people to comprehend, it would probably be a practical necessity. And once the clients began running the retreats *in toto,* there would be no doubt in anyone's mind that the old "hospital" had ceased to exist. The government would also pay the salaries of a certain number of tutors who would be available to clients in the retreat and also the personnel needed to staff the sheltered workshops. This would still be far less expensive than the present system where the government must maintain not only a "medical" staff in mental "hospitals" but an administrative staff as well.

What of the small number of mental "patients" who really have brain diseases? Since there would no longer be any mental "hospitals" where would they go? These people should be cared for in general hospitals if they really have brain diseases. They should be treated in exactly the same way as other truly sick patients are treated. A person with a metabolic disturbance of the brain which we call "acute schizophrenia" would be treated in the same hospital as a person with a metabolic disturbance of the pancreas which we call diabetes. Since there would no longer be any psychiatrists per se, the hospital care of these patients could be handled by general practitioners, internists, and neurologists. The probability that such an arrangement would be satisfactory is indicated by a recent study which showed that general practitioners are equally as competent as psychiatrists in treating "psychiatric inpatients" in a general hospital.[6]

As soon as the "acute schizophrenia" was under medical control, then the patient would be discharged from the hospital. A follow-up outpatient visit would be arranged just as it would be for a patient with diabetes. Since problems of living almost invariably accompany a disease like "schizophrenia," most such patients would be urged by their doctors to contract with a tutor. This could be done independently or through a retreat. Using this resource, the patient could learn how to avoid unnecessary stress which might precipitate recurrence of the disease and how to solve the problems of living which accompany a disease like "schizophrenia." This is equally true for people with diseases like diabetes which tend to recur or become chronic. The division of labor between the doctor and the tutors, then, would be drawn along the line which separates diseases from problems of living. Currently this line is blurred with many doctors spending so much time on patients' problems of living that there is no time left for real diseases. In the case of psychiatrists, it is extreme—we are trained as doctors yet spend most of our practicing lives as teachers. Once psychiatrists cease to exist, the motley assortment of functions will sort themselves rather quickly into either the medical or the educational model.

The prototype of the division being advocated is currently used for a person who has a reading disorder or a person who is blind. The former is seen first by a doctor who treats any medical condition which may be contributing to the reading disorder. The person is then advised to go to a teacher who can teach him to read. Similarly, a blind person is treated first by a doctor who does whatever he can medically, but then the person is tutored by a special teacher to learn how to get along in life.

As was mentioned previously, tutors would be selected for the profession on the basis of their personality characteristics and previous life experience as well as their ability to learn. This should ensure that a broad range of tutors, spanning all socioeconomic and cultural backgrounds, would be available. It would contrast sharply with the present situation where the vast majority of mental "health" professionals are upper class with Anglo-Saxon or Jewish backgrounds. Certainly many tutors would be drawn from the ranks of people who now become psychiatrists, psychologists, anthropologists, sociologists, and social workers; but many others would be individuals who had little formal education but who had the requisite personality characteristics and life experience.

THE EDUCATIONAL CONTRACT

Any person with a problem of living could contract with a tutor to get help with the problem. The contract would always be mutually voluntary. It might be for private tutoring or for tutoring of a group. Since many tutors would have areas of special interest or expertise, a client with a problem would try and find a tutor whose expertise coincided with the client's problem. In addition to matching on the basis of problems and expertise, there would also be an attempt to match on the basis of personality characteristics and world-view. This is important in light of the evidence previously cited that the interaction of personalities of client and tutor is intergral to the learning process. Thus, a liberal, agnostic client would never be paired with a conservative, deeply religious tutor. Such matching could even be computerized. It sounds utopian, but since it is currently tried for dating, it can certainly be tried for learning. Currently much searching goes on by "patients" for a "therapist" who they feel comfortable with, but the searching is random. Computerizing it would produce much better results.

There is reason to believe that matching clients and tutors is important in both "psychotherapy" and education. In the former, one type of "therapist" was found to get better results with inpatient "schizophrenics" whereas another type of therapist did better with outpatient "neurotics."[7] In education, a study showed that students who are relatively well-adjusted desire a nondirective teacher whereas those who are not as well-adjusted want a more directive teacher.[8] Another study

along the same lines showed that "students who are depen-
dent and need structure do significantly better if they have a
teacher who is authoritarian and needs to structure the learning situation."[9] The converse was also found to be true. Perhaps such matching is the wave of the future.

Together the client (or clients) and the tutor would set the
goals of the educational contract. Such goals might include
anything from help with a well-defined problem area (e.g., a
phobia) to a broad mandate to help the person change his life
style. The college student with study problems might want
only to be able to study, the alcoholic might want to stop
drinking, and the boy with low intelligence may want to learn
how to get along without getting into trouble. The tutor may
decide that his client's goals are unrealistic without broadening the areas of inquiry, e.g., that the study problem cannot
be solved without exploring the student's relationship with
his father. The student can then accept this modification of
the goals, or look elsewhere for a tutor who will accept his
more circumscribed goals.

The goals would, of course, be both culture-bound and
class-bound. There would be no expectation that everyone
would want to learn the same thing. People from one subcul-
ture may want to learn how to accept God's will, while people
from another may want to learn how to create a meaning for
life in the absence of God. A college professor may want to
learn why he has been divorced by three wives, while a blue
collar worker may want to learn what he can do about the
tedium of his job.

In a neo-educational model, the goals are always one stage
in an unending continuum. The end of the continuum, complete education, is an unobtainable ideal. Therefore goals are
always intermediate way-stations on the path toward the ideal.
To attain a complete education or self-education is a task for
Sisyphus. Because the goals are regarded in a relative rather
than an absolute sense, however, there would be no talk of
"cures." People learn and they may use what they learn more
or less efficiently; but they are never "cured" unless they are
really sick. The whole medical concept of "cures" for problems
of living would be discarded altogether. Similarly, the sterile

arguments about whether "psychotherapy" really "works" or not would be thrown out and would be replaced by arguments about the educational model. These arguments would focus on how much the person had learned, what kind of a tutor facilitated the learning, and how much the person had been able to carry over from theory to practice.

Another aspect of the educational contract is that of professionalism. How much responsibility will a tutor take for his client? Will he get up at three in the morning if the client calls him? Will he try and stop his client from committing suicide? Within the medical model, the answers to these questions have been relatively easy to obtain by invoking the hoary Hippocratic Oath. What would happen once Hippocrates was no longer available?

First, it should be pointed out that doctors do not have a corner on the market of professionalism. Educators, too, have codes that govern their conduct with their students, though these codes are usually unwritten and are not as well formulated as those in medicine. However, there are certain basic rules that are generally accepted among educators; for example, a teacher should not exploit a student.

It is possible, moreover, to advance these unwritten codes into a more formal document which would guide the conduct of tutors. The exact terms of the code would then be agreed upon by the client and the tutor as part of their initial educational contract. For instance, the general code for all tutors might include such items as the fact that the tutor may not exploit his client under any condition. That would mean that a tutor could not do things like seducing a client or use a client to achieve a political favor. Another possible example might be that the tutor must agree to accept responsibility, within reason, for crises that the client undergoes in the course of his self-education. In other words, if the tutor and client meet on Friday afternoon and the client calls up in panic Friday night, the tutor may not disclaim all responsibility until the following Monday. Self-education should not be conceived of as a nine-to-five job for either the client or the tutor. The exact limits of the responsibility would have to be worked out between them.

Still another part of the general code might include the issue of confidentiality. It might be expected that a tutor would hold confidential all information which he learned during his work with a client. This confidentiality would extend even to a court of law unless released from the contract by the client. It might also extend past the death of the client, i.e., a tutor could not write a book about a famous client he had tutored even after the client had died.

The problem of responsibility for a person who wants to kill himself is a difficult one. The medical model, through its Hippocratic roots, locks the "therapist" into a rather singular position of always having to save the person, even if it means locking the person up "for his own good." The neo-educational model, on the other hand, would be more flexible. One tutor may believe that life is not necessarily the *summum bonum* and that a person who wants to kill himself has that right. Another tutor may believe killing oneself is a mortal sin and not justified under any condition. Both tutors would make their positions clear to a client before the educational contract was signed. The client, of course, would most likely choose a tutor who shared his own point of view.

In the last analysis, tutors would have to be licensed and accredited in order to achieve the needed professionalism. This would be not only a necessity but a vast improvement over the current state of affairs. As things now stand, people with problems of living may be "treated" by a whole range of individuals from highly qualified "psychotherapists" with multiple professional degrees to itinerant soothsayers. In New York State, for example, anybody at all can declare himself to be a "psychotherapist," "psychoanalyst," "hypnotist," "marriage counselor," or "group therapist" as these titles are not protected by laws. There is virtually no regulation of the adequacy of training even for psychiatrists.[10] It is a penetrating commentary on our society that we regulate who may fix a broken faucet but not who may fix a broken marriage.

Thus, by setting up a system of accreditation and licensing, a uniformity would be achieved of who could help people with problems of living. The internecine struggles among psychiatrists, psychologists, social workers, counselors of various sorts, and self-appointed "psychotherapists" would be over, resolved by accrediting tutors to help people and razing the remaining boundaries of the artificial disciplines.

In addition to accreditation and licensing, a system of review and appeal would be needed to maintain professionalism. This might consist of a board composed of *both* tutors and consumers who would review cases of alleged unprofessional conduct brought before it. If a client thought that his tutor had not fulfilled the terms of the contract, he could ask for a review by the board. Some mechanism such as this is necessary to maintain high standards of conduct among any service profession.

A mundane yet very important aspect of the educational contract is the financial aspect. Tutors would be working for money, but who would be responsible for paying them and how much? One possibility is that this could be handled in the same way that general education presently is handled. The state would be responsible for making available to all students a certain level of self-education. This could be accomplished by the courses in behavioral science and self-education taught in public educational institutions. Beyond that point, each individual could purchase further self-education privately either in response to a particular problem or just to enlarge his knowledge. At the national level, funds might be made available for basic research in the behavioral science areas, probably coordinated through the National Institutes of Behavioral Science, a logical successor to the National Institute of Mental Health. There could be separate institutes to study and coordinate training for specific problems of national interest, e.g., violence, alcoholism, and drug addiction.

The question of insurance coverage for problems of mental "illness" presently confronting the insurance industry would be obviated. Three-quarters of the problems which fall into the category of problems of living would not be covered any more than unhappiness or a rainy day is covered by insurance. The other people with true brain diseases would be covered just as diseases of the kidneys and lungs are covered.

A thorny problem is that of the administration of medication. Should tutors ever administer medicine to their clients?

Arguing in the affirmative, one can say it is not very difficult to teach a person how to use psychoactive drugs since a very limited number of them are in use. One psychiatrist claims that "...all the factual material relevant for the effective and practical use of psychoactive drugs could be learned in two weeks by the average intelligent student in the mental health field."[11] Another indication of this is that a computer has been programmed to prescribe psychiatric drugs when symptoms of a patient are fed into it; its agreement with clinical psychiatric judgment has been found to be 84 percent.[12] On the other hand, if tutors used drugs, it might blur the distinction between the medical and the neo-educational model and we would end up right back where we began. This may well militate against tutors prescribing drugs. A final answer to this question will probably have to await actual experience with the neo-educational model.

Tutors would, however, be expected to be alert for signs and symptoms of true brain disease in clients who came to them with problems of living. This alertness could be taught relatively easily during the courses of training as behavioral scientists. In addition, tutors could administer simple pencil and paper screening tests devised to detect organic brain disease; such tests exist and are moderately reliable. All suspicious cases where doubt exists in the tutor's mind would be referred to an internist or neurologist for a definitive examination. With such a procedure, there is no reason to believe that any more cases of true organic brain disease would be mislabeled as problems of living than are presently mistaken by psychiatrists; and these are very few.

All these aspects of the educational contract would have to be worked out by trial and error, of course, once the neo-educational model was instituted. The above are only suggestions for the purposes of illustration and discussion. The final answers to these questions would emerge out of the period of searching as the medical model slowly withers and dies. It is suggested that, following Kuhn's thesis of how models change, we are now entering into such a transition period.

12

People as Human Beings: Legal Implications

THE uniqueness of human beings lies in our self-consciousness. It is this self-consciousness which allows us to be responsible for our actions. Depriving human beings of this responsibility is the ultimate insult, for it consigns us to less-than-human status.

This is exactly what the medical model of human behavior does. It sees human behavior as determined by such things as biochemical predispositions and the experiences of childhood. Human beings in this view become machines determined by forces beyond their control and it is these forces which determine what the person will do. The human, rather than being free, becomes a prisoner of the id and chemicals of the brain. Freud represented this point of view *par excellence* when he described man's behavior as the product of intrapsychic forces, forces which were exerted through a plumber's nightmare of cerebral pipes, valves, gauges, and pressure outlets.

Such a view of human beings ignores our uniqueness—the peculiar arrangement of our brain cells which allows us to contemplate ourselves and our actions. We can assess the effects of past actions and plan the probabilities of future actions. As such, we have a freedom of behavior that is not enjoyed by lower animals.

The medical model deprives us of this freedom of behavior. By viewing us as a machine and our behavior as determined by forces beyond our control, proponents of the medical model have been able to arrive at the idea of nonresponsibility. People who are mentally "ill" are those whose forces have gotten out of control. As such they cannot be held responsible. This leads logically to things like declaring people unfit to stand trial, involuntary confinement, and the insanity defense, a panoply of prejudice and partiality that besmirches our judicial scene.

When the medical model of human behavior is discarded, the concept of nonresponsibility is discarded as well. People become fully responsible for their actions. And since there is no group of people called the mentally "ill," there is no group who can be called not responsible and thereby deprived of their uniqueness as human beings.

The only exceptions to this are the small group of people who have actual brain disease. These people, in some cases, may not be responsible for their behavior. For instance, the man with brain syphilis (who thought his wife was trying to poison him) and the woman with a brain tumor (who had propositioned two men on the street), described in Chapter 10, would not necessarily be responsible for their actions. They may not be responsible because they have an actual disease of their brain which is the overriding determinant of their actions. The brain syphilis and the brain tumor have usurped their freedom of action. This group, however, as mentioned previously, is very small and represents no more than 5 percent of people we refer to as mentally "ill."

The problem remains of what to do about the people we now call "psychotics." Some of these people probably have true brain diseases and some probably do not. All of them have abundant problems of living as well. Examples of such individuals are the last five people described in Chapter 10. Should these people be held responsible for their actions, or are they not responsible?

Within the present limitations of our knowledge about the causes of "schizophrenia" and other forms of "psychosis," we must proceed and assign responsibility on the basis of probability. Probably the two chronically incapacitated individuals described in Chapter 10 (the forty-year-old woman and the middle-aged man) have brain diseases resulting in their being labeled as "chronic schizophrenics." They should not be held responsible for their behavior. Nor probably should the boy who had withdrawn from his family and was hearing voices. He appears to be similar to other people that we call "acute schizophrenics" and may or may not progress to a more chronically incapacitated state. His nonresponsibility would be operative only during his illness and would not carry over once he began to recover.

On the other hand, the woman who thinks that Communists are plotting against her and the man who is "high" and spending all his money probably should be held responsible. They *may* have a form of true brain disease, but then again they may not. Although I know that many other psychiatrists would disagree with the statement, I do not think that either one of them *probably* has a brain disease. Yes, they have unusual thinking patterns, but unusual thinking is not sufficient to deprive people of their civil liberties and basic rights. Six months or 6 years from now, we may know more about how their brains are actually functioning; and at that time, we may be able to say definitely one way or the other. But for the present, we just do not have that kind of knowledge.

The underlying principle which I am utilizing to judge human behavior is the assumption that a person is responsible until it is proven (on the basis of probability at least) that he is not. Human dignity demands that much as a minimum. The object of the laws is to protect people who are truly sick but not to deprive people of their freedom just because they behave or believe strangely by community standards. If we have to err, it is better that we err on the side of human dignity and call too few, rather than too many, people "sick."

One of the most important consequences of accepting these people as responsible is that they will be encouraged to accept that responsibility themselves. It is the same principle as in raising a child—assume that they are going to be responsible and they will usually *be* responsible. As phrased by a psychiatrist in the terms of the medical model:

> ... it must now be clear that the treatment transaction with all its technical and human encounters must have as its major goal helping the patient to assume increasing

responsibility for his feelings, his thoughts, his fantasies, his view of reality, and the conduct of his life. If we look at the assumption of responsibility as the crucial variable in therapy and if we see illness as a position of help-lessness and irresponsibility while health is an existence of independence and responsibility, then therapy must help the patient in that direction.[1]

It should be added at this point that holding all people (except the few with overriding brain disease) responsible for their behavior does not necessarily mean that they will all be punished in the same way for transgressions. A man may steal $100 but he may steal it for quite different reasons; he may steal it because his family is starving, because voices told him to steal it, because someone bet him that he would not dare to, because he needed it to pay off a creditor who was threatening him, or because he wanted to play the horses. In each case, the man is legally responsible for the theft in the sense that he took the money. However, judges and juries will deal with each case quite differently, taking into consideration all the facts and extenuating circumstances. It is at *this* level, not the level of responsibility *per se,* that facts regarding problems of living can be brought into the legal equation. This will be described more fully below.

It should also be clear from what has already been said that all alcohol and narcotics addicts should be held responsible for their actions. This is true, even though technically they may have an acute chemical brain disease (due to alcohol or narcotics) at the time of their action. The important thing is that the brain disease in these cases is *self-induced.* Since they purposefully took the alcohol or narcotics, they become responsible for everything they do while under its influence. The same holds true for individuals who ingest LSD or other mind-altering drugs.

This discussion of the legal responsibility of people formerly called mentally "ill" has an analogy in recent discussions about the "cause" of criminal behavior. In these discussions, there has been speculation that criminal behavior may be "caused" by an XYY chromosome abnormality. The individual born with this abnormality is said to be tall, below average in intelligence, and strongly predisposed to personality deviation and criminality. This, of course, is just a modern-day revival of the "bad seed" theorists of yesteryear. And despite its facade of genetic respectability, the XYY theory is just as demeaning to human beings as saying that a person's behavior is "caused" by the shape of his skull. Such theories rob human beings of their essential humanity by robbing them of their free will. They imply that man is not responsible for his actions because these actions are "caused" by things over which he has no control. As such, they are very similar to the discussions of mentally "ill" people as being not responsible.

THE IMPLICATIONS OF RESPONSIBILITY

When the concept of nonresponsibility is rejected outright, then people who we have called mentally "ill" are given back some of their dignity. They are rescued from their rung on the ladder of life that placed them with lower animals. Thus the very act of declaring people to be responsible can restore some of their self-esteem. Furthermore, it would make it more difficult to discredit their thoughts and achievements. Nobody would write more books trying to prove that Jesus was a "paranoid" because even if it could be proven, it would not change the quality of His thoughts or actions. People called "paranoid" would be no less responsible than people called "republicans" or "Rotarians."

Furthermore, there would be no such thing as depriving a person of his right to stand trial. Everyone would retain this civil liberty as guaranteed by the Constitution and it could not be usurped by a psychiatrist or a judge. The only exception, as mentioned previously, would be people with true brain disease (such as a brain tumor) and then the delay would only be until their medical condition had improved. But these cases are very rare. As one study concluded: "Incompetency to stand trial on the basis of mental illness is rare and is usually quickly responsive to treatment."[2] Brain disease, then, would be put on exactly the same basis as heart disease and kidney disease. To argue that it is unfair to, say, force a "paranoid" to stand trial is to argue only that our system of justice is not perfect. As stated by Szasz:

> No two people are equally capable of defending themselves against criminal charges. Hence, even if some so-

called mental illnesses should impair a person's capacity to defend himself—others, however, might improve it—it would be no more logical not to try a person for this reason than for relative lack of education. Surely, a cleaning woman, accused of political subversion, cannot defend herself as well as a professor of political science. This, however, does not prevent us from trying her.[3]

DANGEROUS TO SELF OR OTHERS

It should not be possible to confine people against their wills in mental "hospitals." If people are held to be universally responsible, then the rationale for such confinement ceases to exist.

Usually people who are confined against their will are said to be not responsible insofar as they are dangerous to themselves or dangerous to others. Regarding the first, I would argue that we are *all* dangerous to ourselves. Each time a man picks up a cigarette or drives too fast, he is dangerous to himself. The difference between these situations and the one in which the man tells you clearly that he wants to kill himself is a difference of degree, not of kind. And in no case do we have the right to call the person not responsible and lock him up until he gives us right answers.

This implies that people have the right to kill themselves if they wish. I believe that this is so. Suicide may be a perfectly rational—and responsible—solution to situations in which people find themselves. We do not generally acknowledge this in our culture because of our Judeo-Christian heritage with its premium on the quantity, rather than the quality, of life. In other cultures, suicide is often considered a perfectly responsible act, sometimes even the *most* responsible act. Socrates increased rather than decreased his dignity by his suicide. We occasionally have glimmerings of this even in our culture, as when an old man with cancer kills himself or when a person sets fire to himself on the lawn of the Pentagon to protest a war he considers unjust. But usually when a person says he wants to kill himself, we just label him as mentally "ill," therefore not responsible, therefore a candidate for the locked mental "ward" until he changes his mind.

This does not mean, however, that we should ignore a person who says that he wants to die. We can and should offer such a person all the resources at our disposal, including immediate attention by a tutor, assessment of the crisis, and an offer of ongoing help in solving whatever the problems are. Usually this is exactly what the person wants, as his suicide threat is really a cry for help. But under no circumstances can we coerce the person to accept the help or confine him involuntarily.

Regarding a person who is adjudged to be "dangerous to others," such a person should be dealt with in a judicial rather than a medical manner. Just as a man who threatens the life of the President can be prosecuted, so a man who threatens the life of others could be prosecuted also. The seriousness of the threat and the relative degree of danger would be up to a judge and jury to decide; it would not be a medical question at all.

Putting such questions back into their proper judicial framework should simultaneously cause the courts to reevaluate the concept of "dangerous to others." What is the relative danger to others, for instance, of a "paranoid" who thinks his neighbors are plotting against him and an alcoholic with three drunken-driving arrests? And is a "voyeur" more dangerous to others than an armed robber? These are the questions that need asking. Currently, however, we do not ask them but merely consign a group of people, who we label mentally "ill," to indeterminate sentences in mental "hospitals" on the grounds that they are "dangerous to others." People who are really dangerous to others should be legally (not medically) confined in direct proportion to the actual magnitude of the danger.

If any other reasons are needed to remove "dangerous" persons from the realm of medicine and return them to law, it might be added that psychiatrists are very poor predictors of human behavior. In studies of people who are incarcerated, it has been shown that psychiatrists consistently overpredict antisocial behavior.[4] As mentioned in Chapter 5, it has also been shown that people incarcerated as mentally "ill" are no more dangerous when released than anyone else in the general population.

THE INSANITY DEFENSE

If psychiatry dies there will be no more "insanity." And if there is no "insanity," then there will be no insanity defense. This is as it should be and would follow logically from what has been said previously about this judicial embarrassment.

If there was no insanity defense, then a person would never be found "not guilty by reason of insanity." The person would either be guilty or not guilty. There would be no such person as a psychiatrist in the courtroom at all at this stage. Psychiatrists really have no more right to decide who is guilty and not guilty than does the Good Humor man.

It would be at the next stage of the procedure—the sentencing—that a behavioral scientist might come into the judicial picture as an expert witness. The question at this stage is not one of guilt but rather one of degree of responsibility. All persons found guilty are assumed to be responsible to some degree, but the degree may vary widely.

To return to the example cited earlier, the man who steals $100 because his family is starving is likely to be given a different sentence than the man who steals $100 to play the horses; and he in turn will be sentenced differently than the man who steals $100 because voices told him to do so. Furthermore, a judge may take into consideration such extenuating circumstances as the fact that the man's father had died the previous week or that the man belongs to a fundamentalist religious sect which firmly believes that the world is going to end in one week.

A behavioral scientist, if he belongs in court at all, belongs there as a witness at the stage of sentencing. He could introduce whatever knowledge he has regarding what the voices told the man, just as he could testify about the duress the man had been under at work or any other circumstances which might have influenced the man's behavior. In this role, the behavioral scientist would simply try and inform the judge and jury about the circumstances that existed at the time of the crime in order to help them assess the degree of responsibility and relative liability of the man. It should also be added that when our system of education is modified so as to include the science of human behavior as an integral part of the curriculum, then judges and juries will have a much better under-standing of human behavior to begin with, even without a behavioral scientist in the courtroom as an expert witness.

It should also be recognized that the role of a behavioral scientist in the courtroom at the stage of sentencing would be a partisan one. He would be testifying for either one side or the other—in other words, to show that the man's responsibility was diminished because of certain circumstances (defense) or to show that the circumstances surrounding the crime were not important (prosecution). The current courtroom scene with os-tensibly nonpartisan psychiatrists and psychologists arguing with each other is a farce. If behavioral scientists come into the courtroom at all, they should come clearly labeled as a witness for either the defense or the prosecution. Such a scheme has been previously suggested by Szasz.[5]

Most importantly, however, the behavioral scientist would not be there at all until the stage of sentencing. He would be completely excluded from the part of the trial in which guilt was determined. It is important that we be able to learn from the long dreary history of the psychiatrist in the courtroom. As summarized by Professor Dershowitz of Harvard, one of the most astute observers of the scene:

> It is a discouraging history of usurpation and abdication: of an expert being summoned for a limited purpose, as-suming his own indispensability, and then persuading the law to ask the critical questions in terms which make him more comfortable and his testimony more relevant. The upshot has been to make the psychiatrist's testimony more relevant to the questions posed, but to make the questions themselves less relevant to the purpose of the law.[6]

It has been encouraging to see the beginning of psychiatric reform in the judiciary in the past few years. It was a court decision in Alabama which declared that mental "patients" have a right to "treatment."[7] A court in New York said that mental "patients" must be paid for labor which they perform while being confined in "hospitals" and a court in Florida awarded damages to a "patient" who had been held involunta-rily and not properly "treated."[8] These court cases, just the tip of a legal iceberg, have been immeasurably helped along by organizations such as the Center for Law and Social Policy in Washington, the American Civil Liberties Union, the National Council on the Rights of the Mentally Impaired, and the Association for the Abolition of Involuntary Mental Hospitalization.

THE STUNTED GROWTH OF LAW

The most important ramifications in seeing people as human beings—and therefore as responsible—may be on the field of law itself. It is a field whose current methodologies have produced the near bankruptcy of justice and whose institutions for corrections have produced only more criminality. It is a field badly in need of basic reform.

One of the impediments to this reform, I would submit, has been the existence of psychiatry. By lobbying for the nonresponsibility of a class of individuals called the mentally "ill," psychiatry has contributed large amounts of mud to the clear stream of reason. Psychiatrists have been allowed to gradually assume increasing responsibility for deciding who can stand trial and, once on trial, who is guilty. The decision-making process has become increasingly medical and decreasingly judicial: "So effective has been the incursion of the therapeutic state into the old penal system that less than half of the American population may now be subject to the sanctions of criminal law."

But it has been a mutually convenient affair. By being able to consign a large number of individuals to psychiatry, the law has not had to deal with them. The man who stands on the street corner talking to himself, the alcoholic sleeping in an alley, the man who peeps into other people's windows, the woman who threatens to burn down her neighbor's house—these and many more can be taken by the policeman and dumped on the doorstep of his friendly local psychiatrist. The psychiatrist in turn sends them to the state hospital for 72 hours of "observation." Make no mistake, if psychiatry were abolished, the law enforcement officials who benefit from the present psychiatric dumping ground would be very unhappy.

The immediate effect of the abolition of psychiatry would be to put all those who we presently label mentally "ill" back into the courts. Although this might cause some initial chaos, in the long run it would help force the legal profession to reform itself. Everyone can agree that we need to punish illegal behavior; what we need more discussions of is what constitutes illegal behavior. Compare, for instance, the threat to society posed by a woman who threatens her neighbor and a corporation which threatens the water supply to a city by dumping pollutants. Compare a man who stands on the corner talking to himself with a slumlord who paints his apartments with leaded paint. Compare a "manic" who spends money he does not have with a businessman who spends money on his expense account. Compare a "psychopath" who tries to deceive people with an advertising company which tries to deceive people. When the legal profession begins to ask itself such questions, then the process of reform will begin. But the questions will not be asked as long as one category of people whose behavior is deviant are labeled as "sick" and consigned to medical incarceration.

Similarly, the institutions of the legal field, the jails and prisons, need to be reformed. What is their purpose supposed to be? Is it to protect other members of society from personal injury? In that case, only 10 or 15 percent of the individuals in prisons need to be there; the rest are car thieves, bad check cashers, alcoholics, drug addicts, and the like. Is the purpose to punish people who break laws and deter future law-breaking? In that case, prisons probably produce as much future criminal activity as they deter by exposing young law-breakers to the company and methods of the more experienced. Is the purpose to teach and rehabilitate individuals? In that case, why are there not more open institutions, home furloughs, halfway houses, and education of the inmates on problems of living? These are questions that must be asked and answered directly, not evaded by redefining people as mentally "ill" and incarcerating them in other kinds of institutions.

In the proposal to abolish psychiatry, the part which is probably most difficult to accept is that which runs counter to recent attempts to humanize the law. These attempts have relied on shifting an increasing amount of deviant behavior to the province of psychiatry. Thus, the reformers would take deviant behavior such as alcoholism and narcotics addiction away from the system of justice and place them instead in the hands of medicine. This is just one phase of the ongoing trend toward defining more and more deviant behavior as mental "illness" and thus shifting the individuals from prisons to "hospitals."

It is difficult to disagree with this because it is being done for the best of reasons—to get more humane "treatment" for these individuals. However, many mistakes have been made for the best of reasons and I believe that this trend is a major mistake. It not only requires that all these individuals be defined as mentally "ill" (with all its implications and complications), but it also permits the legal field to be excused from having to accommodate these individuals (with its implied reform). Thus the attempts to humanize the law by removing from its jurisdiction increasing number of individuals is a failure. It is the wrong thing done for the right reason. It looks good on the outside, but really is like a candy apple that is full of worms.

13
Behavioral Scientists in the Community

WHEN psychiatrists go out into the community, they inevitably follow the road to psychiatric fascism. This, as we saw in Chapter 7, is inherent in the medical model. The community activity of psychiatrists is aimed at preventing disease; so logically they must take whatever steps are necessary in the name of public health.

When behavioral scientists go out into the community, they need not follow this road. They would go not as physicians to prevent disease but as experts in human behavior. And as such, they should be given no more power over other peoples' lives than a plumber or a television repairman. Their power would be only the power to advise and persuade, never to order or coerce.

The settings in which behavioral scientists might work are very broad. They might include everything from retreats and orphanages to urban institutes and the Department of Defense to radio call-in shows. Let us take a brief look at some of the jobs that behavioral scientists might be doing. They include, among others, all the jobs now being done by psychiatrists, clinical psychologists, applied anthropologists, sociologists, and social workers. When individuals assuming these traditional pigeon-holed roles act as true behavioral scientists, they do so in spite of, not because of, their training.

First, the behavioral scientists as tutors would certainly be working at retreats. They would be experts on human behavior and, as such, could help either individuals or groups. Similarly, they might work as tutors at places called Institutes

for Human Problems and other like-sounding edifices where
people could contract to come and get private tutoring. These
places would be human service centers and logical successors
to community mental "health" centers. Some behavioral scientists would probably also open private offices as tutors.

Many behavioral scientists would undoubtedly want to
specialize in certain kinds of problems of living. Groups of
such behavioral scientists practicing together might operate
like Berlitz—your own tutor for whatever problem of living
you wanted to try to solve. Such specialties might include
things like marriage problems, sexual problems, alcoholism,
drug addiction, and depression.

To show how such an expert would differ from the psychiatrists, psychologists, anthropologists, sociologists, or social
workers who presently exist, let us take sexual problems as an
example. A *real* behavioral scientist in this field would be an
expert on such things as how people express sexual feelings
and achieve sexual satisfaction, how this is done in other cultures, the effects of pornography, and how sex education
should be taught. Included in the person's training would
have been the study of research findings on sexual problems
and experiences working with individuals with such problems. The result would be a behavioral scientist who was an
expert in this field. No such person presently exists except for
a handful who are self-taught. This has become painfully evident each time, for instance, a school board summons a psychiatrist to consult on how sex education should be taught in
the school. The psychiatrist's training has included nothing
about sex education. Furthermore, his knowledge of sex and
schools may well be limited to his personal experience, the
oedipal complex, and a patient he once had with school problems. In short, his consultation provides very little expertise.
It is really quite remarkable, and pathetic, that we do not
have real experts in such things as sexual problems. The
death of psychiatry and the emergence of behavioral scientists would help rectify this situation.

Another field in which behavioral scientists might become
specialized is that of antisocial activity. This field is currently
a mass of confusion in which law enforcement officers, correc-

tion officers, lawyers, social workers, clinical psychologists, and sociologists each claim, like the blind men describing an elephant, to have hold of the most important part. Psychiatrists, it should be added, are conspicuously absent from the scene except to come into the courtroom and declare an offender "sick." A behavioral scientist who specialized in antisocial behavior would become an expert on everything known about its antecedents and manifestations. He might try to assess the biological and genetic components, study the relationship of early childhood experiences to such activity, and spend many hours working with adolescents and young adults who were acting antisocially. He might do cross-cultural studies to try and identify the cultural factors which predispose toward antisocial behavior and he would be knowledgeable on the social causes of such behavior.

It should be clearly pointed out, however, that a behavioral scientist who specialized in antisocial activity would not infringe upon law enforcement functions *per se.* He would not be allowed to participate in the apprehension of law breakers, their trial, or their punishment. These traditional judicial functions would remain clearly under the jurisdiction of law enforcement officials. The behavioral scientist *would* participate in activities related to influencing the antecedents of antisocial activity, e.g., he might lobby for gun control or for decreasing violence in children's television programs. He would also be deeply involved in the rehabilitation of offenders once they had passed through the judicial system of trial and punishment. By making a clear distinction between the goals of law enforcement (punishment of offenders and protection of society) and those of behavioral science and education (education and rehabilitation of offenders), the dilemmas of the contemporary scene—expecting one system to both punish and rehabilitate—could be avoided. Trying to make a single person do both of these things is like trying to conceive two-headed children and the end product in both cases is a spontaneous abortion.

There is one other aspect of law enforcement work in which behavioral scientists could provide assistance. This is the vast amount of law enforcement officials' time which is occupied in trying to mediate or solve problems of living. It is estimated that up to 90 percent of calls for police service do not involve violations of laws but rather problems of living. These calls typically include such things as domestic arguments, runaway children, and complaints of bizarre behavior by neighbors. Furthermore, one-half of all arrests are for drunkenness, disorderly conduct, gambling, vagrancy, and minor sexual violations.[1] Many of these calls could be referred to a behavioral scientist when they do not involve a violation of the law. The end result might be a group of behavioral scientists who operate out of a human service center and respond to such calls. They might be likened to meter maids for human problems except that they would not be under the jurisdiction of the police. And law enforcement officials, consequently, would be freed to respond only to those cases in which a law had been violated.

Another example of an area in which behavioral scientists might specialize is that of urban problems. A behavioral scientist in this field would work with the behavioral consequences of people living together in cities. The problem of crowding and the need for "life-space" would be one concern, as would the territoriality of individuals and ethnic groups. Such a behavioral scientist would also work extensively on the problems of intergroup relations, ethnicity, the behavioral effects of poverty, and mass violence. In addition to working with individuals and groups who were having problems of living in these areas, he might consult with city planners, architects, the housing authority, and the Department of Welfare.

Behavioral scientists would probably also be employed by industries in the same way as industrial psychologists and psychiatrists presently are. They could advise on employer-employee relations and offer both individual and group tutoring. They would be experts on how people can satisfy human needs within a large organization and would deal with problems such as what happens to a person's self-esteem when he becomes part of an assembly line process. They would also explore such problem areas as the effect of increasing leisure (and decreasing work) as industrial workweeks are reduced to fewer and fewer hours.

Still another area in which behavioral scientists might specialize is international problems. Some subjects which such a person might be an expert on are the effects of rapid technological development, cultural change, intergroup conflict and methods of its reduction, the relativity of cultural values, and the concept of national character. Such a behavioral scientist might work abroad in foreign assistance programs or at home in the State Department or the Department of Defense. The need for behavioral scientists in the last organization is reflected by the fact that recently there were only 3 people with backgrounds in behavioral sciences among the 150 people working in the planning and evaluation section (the "think tank") of the Pentagon. Small wonder that our foreign policy has been a series of blunders with little regard shown for the human factors in the equation.

This last point leads to the problem of the politicization of behavioral scientists. Purists in present behavioral science disciplines often argue that behavioral scientists, *qua* scientists, have no business becoming involved in the political process. The implication is that the political process is tainted and that it is somehow beneath the dignity of a true scientist.

In fact, this is both elitist and erroneous. The political process is the decision-making process. Unless and until behavioral scientists participate in it, they must not expect it to incorporate behavioral concepts to any large degree. For instance, as long as foreign policy decisions are made exclusively by economists, lawyers, and political scientists, then one must expect the decisions to reflect predominately economic, legal, and political considerations. Behavioral scientists must be willing to come out of their oaken libraries and enter into the fray. Of course, their data will be "used" for political purposes—and it should be "used"—just as economic data is "used." But in the process of being "used," it will add the critical factor of human behavior to the decision-making equation. Behavioral scientists will never play a determining role in political decisions, but they can play *some* role if they are willing to enter into the public arena and fight for the values which they believe are important.

The net effect of having behavioral scientists enter into the community, not as medical men but as educators and problem solvers, would be an increased humanization of decision making. It is really quite incredible that we do not have any true behavioral scientists except the handful who have emerged, self-taught, by departing from their narrow disciplinary base. Until psychiatry dies, a strong cadre of true behavioral scientists is not likely to emerge. Once they do, however, then possibly we can promote the conservation of human resources with as much vigor as we promote the conservation of natural resources.

14
Conclusions:
Psychiatry as a Platypus

PSYCHIATRY is like the platypus. This mammal, found only in Australia and Tasmania, is a shy, furry creature with web feet and a broad duck bill that appears totally out of proportion to its body. It is an absurd animal. It is also an evolutionary dead end, unable to defend itself and headed toward extinction. From the historical point of view, it was a clear improvement over the reptile; however, we can now see that it was a false lead on the mammalian evolutionary tree and that the main limb was one of the placentals which evolved through the moles and the hedgehogs to become larger mammals.

Evolutionary dead ends like the platypus and psychiatry play a function, however. By evolving as far as they are able, we can see how well they function and so better select the main evolutionary limb. In the case of mammals, this turned out to be the placentals. In the case of psychiatry, we do not yet know what it will be. I have suggested the limb of education as a possibility. Searching for the main limb and discarding dead ends is what evolution is all about. We may not know for many years what the best choice actually is. We do know, however, that we must continue to try new models. This is the fundamental rule of our biological and institutional existence—adapt or abdicate.

In discussing the death of psychiatry, I have been describing an historical and evolutionary event which is, I believe, currently in progress. And insofar as psychiatry's death may eventually lead to better human services for those members of our society who need them (and most of us do), then I am sympathetic with it. To minimize misconceptions about what I have or have not advocated, it may be useful to briefly summarize. One of the most effective tricks which our minds play on us is to not understand things which we do *not want* to understand. It affords us the illusion of equilibrium on a listing ship and acts as a life preserver for those who fear drowning when asked to rethink an idea or a belief.

I have said that the medical model of human behavior should be banished to the realm of the dodo bird and the dinosaur. When its medical rhetoric is followed to its logical conclusion, it ends up in the land of the absurd. To call people who have problems with their behavior "diseased" is to activate connotations and complications which can be very destructive. The various parts of the disease model—classification, causes, diagnosis, doctors, hospitals, therapies, cure, and nonresponsibility—have been systematically examined to illustrate this. Diseases are something we have, behavior is something we do.

In place of the medical model, I have proposed an educational model. It would utilize people chosen partly for their personality characteristics (tutors) and train them broadly in the behavioral sciences. The boundaries between psychiatry, psychology, anthropology, sociology, and the other artificial disciplines would be abolished as would the disciplines themselves. Present practitioners of these disciplines would become behavioral scientists and in the case of psychiatry some would return to being neurologists. Expertise would be along behavioral lines (e.g., aggressive, sexual) rather than along antecedents-of-the-behavior lines (e.g., anthropology, psychology). The emphasis would be on teaching people about their throughts, feelings, and behavior, not on treating their anatomy.

I have not, therefore, said that the functions performed by psychiatry should die, but rather that the discipline is dying and should die. This is not only inevitable but constructive; for once it dies, its functions can then be reallocated in a more rational way.

I do not claim to have final answers to all the problems I have raised. Perhaps such answers will be found if sufficient discussion can be provoked. My overwhelming hope is that we may begin the process of recategorization. It is as if we have one hundred balls in a psychiatric box. The first five we saw were red (the people with organic brain disease) so we declared that all the balls must be red. But if we look again we can see that the next seventy-five balls are blue (the people with problems of living). The remaining twenty balls seem to be shades of intermediate colors and will require closer examination to make a final assignment. But just because the last ball cannot be definitely and finally assigned does not mean that we have to continue calling all hundred balls red. Yet this is what we are presently doing in psychiatry.

Change will not come easily. In this case, the change involves not only the institution of psychiatry but the whole model of how human behavior is viewed. Psychiatry and the medical model are not likely to just pass out of existence overnight. Rather we will continue to pass through the crises described by Kuhn in *The Structure of Scientific Revolutions.*[1] In the process of passing through these crises, many arguments will be raised in defense of psychiatry and the medical model. It is useful to briefly review some of the arguments:

1. *Departure from the medical model is retrogressive; it is a return to the past.* It should be remembered that the medical model replaced the theological model of human behavior. Devils and demons were thought to be the cause of strange behavior not too many years ago and the minister or priest was in charge of driving them out. When more conservative methods failed, then the person so afflicted was burned at the stake "for his own good." Psychiatry replaced the devils and demons with brain biochemistry and id and doctors were put in charge of the afflicted. This was no small advance. To abandon the medical model, however, does not mean that we must regress to a theological model. We can instead progress to an educational model. In terms of the people who exhibit strange behavior, we would be moving from a theological model (exorcising the devils) to a medical model (curing the disease) to an educational model (teaching them why they do it). Thus, it is progressive rather than regressive.

2. *Departure from the medical model will displease determinists as opposed to those of us who assume that people have free will.* Many of the advances wrought by the behavioral sci-

ences in this century have been strongly supportive of seeing man's behavior as determined by inside (e.g., Freudian) and outside (e.g., cultural) forces. From these advances, many people have concluded that man's behavior generally is determined and that he does not have free will. This conclusion I specifically disavow. While agreeing that man's choices may be quite restricted at times, I have never met, nor can I imagine, an individual who did not have some degree of free will. Because of the unique twist of our cerebral circuit, the human animal can contemplate himself and, as such, become aware of the forces trying to determine his behavior. No other animal except possibly the porpoise has this ability. In this cerebral circuit of self-reflection, our ultimate free will is embedded in cement and it cannot be removed. Even the poorest, most deprived ghetto resident, the subject of all kinds of determining forces, never completely succumbs to them. Rather he chooses. His choices may be to try and make it legally, or illegally, or to shoot heroin, or to shoot a policeman, or to just float off a rooftop; but he chooses. And if we say that he has no choices, no free will, but rather that his behavior is determined, then we are removing his remaining human dignity. For then even his act of protest against society becomes an act determined by outside forces for which he is not responsible. No, I see man as responsible for his ultimate behavior and this is an explicit assumption of my recommendations in this book.

3. *Departure from the medical model will increase the mind-body dualism.* Defenders of the medical model will argue that psychiatry has broken down the traditional dichotomy between mind and body. It has, they will maintain, made us aware of how important the mind is in all diseases of the body. If the medical model is abandoned, will we not revert to the previous state of affairs? In fact, we will and should. The mind-body dualism is nonsense, as was shown, for mind is the activity of the brain. Everyone will agree that the brain influences all behavior, but that is not to say that all strange behavior must be thought of as brain disease. And to abandon the medical model does not mean that doctors cannot treat the whole person; they can treat the person's diseases and then teach him about as many of his problems of living as they feel comfort-

able teaching. However, they will "treat" only true diseases—the rest of the activity would be called "teaching."

4. *Departure from the medical model will decrease the humaneness with which we "treat" those who are mentally "ill."* Humanitarian motivation was and continues to be one of the pillars of the medical model. The image of Pinel striking the chains off mental "patients" and setting them free is at the very heart of psychiatry. Psychiatrists readily invoke this image when criticized and contrast the humaneness of medical "treatment" with the former plight of mental "patients" in prisons and poorhouses. This is all true in theory but in practice the image shatters. A visit to a state "hospital" should convince any skeptic. We herd thousands of people into these institutions as if the people were human factory rejects; our rationalization is that they are mentally "sick." This pejorative label ensures that they must pay for their food and shelter with the remainder of their self-esteem. It is a high price and makes one wonder just how humane the medical model really is.

5. *Departure from the medical model will be threatening to people.* If medical terminology is abandoned, people will have to redefine their behavior. An alcoholic or homosexual or depressed person will not be able to take refuge behind a medical label which conveys an illusion of explanation; rather, each will have to assess their own behavior as a function of how they have learned to behave. Moreover, if behavioral science ever became really popular, it would be even more threatening. Children might ask their parents why they always sleep in separate bedrooms or ask their gym teacher why he always takes his shower with the youngest boys. It *is* far less threatening to leave human behavior in the realm of "diseases."

6. *Departure from the medical model will be economically disadvantageous to psychiatrists and drug companies.* This is perfectly true and a major reason why psychiatry is resistant to change. If mental "illness" was redefined as problems of living and opened up as a valid domain for large numbers of behavioral scientists, the salaries presently commanded by psychiatrists would drop like the leaves in the autumn. Since the activity of the behavioral scientists would be educational in nature, it might be expected that the ultimate salary scale would level out in the vicinity of that for the teaching profes-

sion. This would not make any behavioral scientist wealthy; but like other teachers, he would be partially compensated by the intellectual and humanitarian rewards of his work.

Departure from the medical model would also be economically disadvantageous to drug companies. These companies, whose profit margins have been among the highest of any United States industry, have been strong supporters of the medicalization of human behavior. For insofar as human behavior is seen as "disease," then it can theoretically be "cured" by drugs. Thus advertisements for tranquilizers promote them as "curing" the anxiety of such normal life situations as a small child going to school, a young adult going to college, or a parent whose child is getting married. Drug companies have been primarily responsible for our emergence as a drugged society, popping pills for anything and everything. Naturally, these companies would be expected to fiercely resist any de-medicalization of behavior, for it might infringe on their profits.

7. *Departure from the medical model will change the status quo.* This is the ultimate argument of many who would hang on to the medical model. It is the plaintive cry of those who would, like Linus, drag their comfortable old medical model through life with them because it is tradition. As stated by one psychiatrist:

> Well, where are we going? Does not our greatest usefulness and our safety come from adhering rather strictly to medicine, the discipline that nurtured us? I believe so. At present, the "Medical Model" of treatment is under attack by "therapists" of every shade and description. We must have a secure base of operations, a harbor we can depend upon when the winds of social change blow this way and that; and it does seem that medicine is that harbor, for no matter to what heights man's spirit and intentions may soar, he will still be trammeled with a body, and no matter what his status he will have emotional illnesses.[2]

But such exhortations have not relieved the underlying discomfiture which may psychiatrists have felt with the medical model. And commanding all hands to hold to their battle stations is rather ineffectual once the ship starts to go down. We have entered into the period of crises when the old model, the medical model, is being perceived increasingly as inadequate. "Many psychiatrists have had, at least to some degree, the unsettling and bewildering feeling that what they have been doing has been largely worthless and that the premises on which they have based their professional lives were partly fraudulent."[3] Certainly it is easier to maintain the *status quo* than to strike out in new directions and to conceptualize new models. To maintain the *status quo* in the face of facts which do not fit, however, is to resist evolution. It is to follow the platypus. And tradition by itself is a tether on the neck of progress; it is the irrational maintenance of the *status quo* by those who have the advantage.

In the face of this criticism of the medical model, it is important to remind ourselves again what the medical model has accomplished. It moved human behavior out of the devils-and-demons period and injected the theory of humane care for those whose behavior deviates from our own.

Psychoanalysis in particular has made us aware of the basically educational nature of our profession. And because of the influence of psychoanalysis in the United States, this is probably the only Western country which could actually try out an educational model. Most countries in Western and Eastern Europe have continued to see mental "patients" in a much more rigid medical framework than we have. Our efforts to include ever-increasing amounts of human behavior in the medical model has put us, paradoxically, at the forefront to reform the whole system of how we classify and modify human behavior. It is in our country that "the Americanization of the unconscious"[4] has taken place and consequently we are probably the only country which can now explore new models for dealing with problems of human behavior. We appear to have a broad general awareness that deviant behavior is not usually brain "disease"; now we need the courage to follow our awareness and common sense to their logical conclusions.

In the final analysis, we must abandon the medical model of human behavior and allow psychiatry to die because the medical model does not fulfill our needs. Medicine is adequate for understanding human tissues but we need a model for understanding human issues. The major threats to our existence are no longer intracellular and intercellular but rather intrapersonal and interpersonal. We are the generation of Auschwitz, where 2,000 people a day were purposefully killed every day for 4½ years. Have we gone anywhere since Attilla the Hun? Yes, we have improved our science and technology for such killing. We have improved our gross national product and controlled the world's markets and exploited other people. Is this civilization? No, progress involves a society's concern for its members and the value that it attaches to each individual life. This is the true index of civilization. The rest is just existence.

Now that we have explored the dark side of the moon, perhaps we can explore the dark side of our minds. We must learn to cultivate better interpersonal relationships as effectively as we have learned to cultivate better wheat, to conserve human resources as well as natural resources. In order to do this, we need to synthesize our knowledge of human behavior and make it available to everyone. Earthquakes and diseases are no longer our biggest enemies; rather, human behavior is. In light of this, it seems incredible that we have not yet learned to train true behavioral scientists. Psychiatry, by fragmenting a large portion of human behavior off into a medical corner, stands as a major impediment to this development.

The death of psychiatry, then, is not a negative event. It is part of the natural evolution of institutions. And it carries within it, seeds for the birth of an integrated behavioral science.

Notes

CHAPTER 1

1. T. S. Kuhn, *The Structure of Scientific Revolutions* (Chicago: University of Chicago Press, 1962).
2. S. J. Fox, *Science and Justice: The Massachusetts Witchcraft Trials* (Baltimore: Johns Hopkins Press, 1968).

CHAPTER 2

1. G. Zilboorg and G. W. Henry, *A History of Medical Psychology* (New York: Norton, 1941), p. 229.
2. Ibid., pp. 519-521.
3. M. Foucault, *Madness and Civilization: A History of Insanity in the Age of Reason* (New York: Random House, 1965). See also: T. S. Szasz, *The Manufacture of Madness: A Comparative Study of the Inquisition and the Mental Health Movement* (New York: Dell, 1970).
4. M. P. Dumont and C. K. Aldrich, "Family Care After a Thousand Years—A Crisis in the Tradition of St. Dymphna," *American Journal of Psychiatry* 119(2):116-121 (August 1962).
5. Foucault, *Madness and Civilization*, p. 216.
6. S. Freud, *Autobiography* (New York: Norton, 1935).
7. F. G. Alexander and S. J. Selesnick, *The History of Psychiatry* (New York: Harper and Row, 1966), p. 152.
8. I. Galdston, ed., *Historic Derivations of Modern Psychiatry* (New York: McGraw-Hill, 1967), p. 105.
9. Alexander and Selesnick, *The History of Psychiatry*, p. 13.

10. Galdston, *Historic Derivations of Modern Psychiatry*; Szasz claims that this view of Weyer is incorrect. See: Szasz, *The Manufacture of Madness*, p. 12.
11. Ibid., p. 168.
12. Ibid.
13. Freud, *Autobiography*.
14. E. Jones, *The Life and Work of Sigmund Freud* (New York: Basic Books, 1955).
15. F. Field, *The Last Days of Mankind: Karl Kraus and His Vienna* (New York: St. Martin's Press, 1967).
16. Jones, *The Life and Work of Sigmund Freud*, p. 27.
17. Ibid., p. 40.
18. Ibid., p. 28.
19. Freud, *Autobiography*.
20. Ibid.
21. Jones, *The Life and Work of Sigmund Freud*, p. 34.
22. Szasz gives an extensive account of these differences: T. S. Szasz, *The Myth of Mental Illness* (New York: Harper and Row, 1961).
23. G. Serban, "Freudian Man Versus Existential Man," *Archives of General Psychiatry* 17:598-607 (November 1967).
24. Ibid.; and J. R. Barclay, "Franz Brentano and Sigmund Freud," *Journal of Existentialism* 5(17):1-36, 1964.
25. Galdston, *Historic Derivations of Modern Psychiatry*.
26. Jones, *The Life and Work of Sigmund Freud*.
27. According to a recent report, there is now once again an increasing sentiment among psychoanalysts in the United States to admit lay analysts. It is related to the decrease in medical applicants to the analytic training institutes. It will be interesting to see

whether a reversal of policy occurs, which, if it does, will further undermine the medical model. See: "Analyst Sees Young MD's Taking 'Activist Approach'," *Psychiatric News* February 1970).

28. Jones, *The Life and Work of Sigmund Freud*, p. 27.

29. H. S. Hughes, *Consciousness and Society: The Reorientation of European Social Thought 1890-1930* (New York: Knopf, 1958).

30. Jones, *The Life and Work of Sigmund Freud*, 3:287.

31. Ibid., p. 297.

32. Ibid., p. 301.

33. Ibid., p. 289.

34. Ibid.

CHAPTER 3

1. E. F. Torrey, *The Mind Game: Witchdoctors and Psychiatrists* (New York: Emerson Hall, 1972).

2. F. C. Redlich and D. X. Freedman, *The Theory and Practice of Psychiatry* (New York: Basic Books, 1966), p. 277. See also: T. Freeman, "The Learning Component in the Dynamic Psychotherapeutic Situation," in *The Role of Learning in Psychotherapy*, ed., R. Porter (Boston: Little, Brown, 1968).

3. L. Krasner, "Assessment of Token Economy Programmes in Psychiatric Hospitals," in *The Role of Learning in Psychotherapy*, ed., R. Porter.

4. J. P. Campbell and M. D. Dunnette, "Effectiveness of T-Group Experiences in Managerial Training and Development," *Psychological Bulletin* 70(2):73-104 (1968).

5. I. D. Yalom, *The Theory and Practice of Group Psychotherapy* (New York: Basic Books, 1970).

6. R. May, "The Existential Approach," in *American Handbook of Psychiatry*, ed., S. Arieti (New York: Basic Books, 1959), 2:1357.

7. A. Ellis, "Rational-Emotive Psychotherapy," in *Counseling and Psychotherapy: An Overview*, ed., D. S. Arbuckle (New York: McGraw-Hill, 1967).

8. G. Caplan and H. Grunebaum, "Perspectives on Primary Prevention," *Archives of General Psychiatry* 17:331-346, 1967.

9. F. J. Van Rheenen, E. F. Torrey and H. A. Katchadourian, "Preventive Psychiatry: Group Work with Foreign Students" (Presented at the Annual Meeting of the American Psychiatric Association, Washington, D.C., 1971).

10. E. Berne, *Games People Play: The Psychology of Human Relationships* (New York: Grove Press, 1964).

11. H. C. Potter and G. T. Stanton, "Money Management and Mental Health," *American Journal of Psychotherapy* 24(1):79-91, 1970.

12. M. Brown, "The New Body Psychotherapies," *Psychotherapy* 10(2):98-116, 1973.

13. M. Shephard, *The Love Treatment: Sexual Intimacy Between Patients and Psychotherapists* (New York: Paperback Library, 1972).

14. E. R. Hilgard, *Theories of Learning*, 2d. ed. (New York: Appleton-Century-Crofts, 1956).

15. R. H. Woody, "Toward a Rationale for Psychobehavioral Therapy," *Archives of General Psychiatry* 19:197-204, 1968.

16. R. Porter, ed., *The Role of Learning in Psychotherapy* (Boston: Little, Brown, 1968).

CHAPTER 4

1. G. Ryle, *The Concept of Mind* (Oxford: Hutchinson's University Press, 1948).

2. T. S. Szasz, *The Myth of Mental Illness* (New York: Harper and Row, 1961).

3. T. R. Sarbin, "On the Futility of the Proposition that Some People Be Labeled 'Mentally Ill'," *Journal of Consulting Psychology* 31:447-453, 1967.

4. *New York Times*, October 17, 1969.

5. P. V. Lemkau, "Prevention in Psychiatry," *American Journal of Public Health* 55(4):554-560, 1965.

6. For an extensive analysis of early attempts to classify "mental disease," see the appendix of: K. Menninger, *The Vital Balance* (New York: Viking Press, 1963).

7. K. Menninger, "Sheer Verbal Mickey Mouse," *International Journal of Psychiatry* 7(6):415, 1969.

8. S. M. Finch, "Nomenclature for Children's Mental Disorders Need Improvement," *International Journal of Psychiatry* 7(6):415, 1969.

9. B. Jackson, "Reflections on DSM-II," *International Journal of Psychiatry* 7(6):385-392, 1969.

10. D. Train, "They Trained Us To Forget We Were Doctors," *Hospital Physician*, pp. 86-95, November 1968.

11. *San Francisco Chronicle* articles on case, March 31-April 30, 1970. The press named the case "The Cable Car Named Desire."

12. F. Wiseman, "Psychiatry and Law: Use and Abuse of Psychiatry in a Murder Case," *American Journal of Psychiatry*, 118:289-299, 1961.

13. S. R. Goldsmith and A. J. Mandell, "The Dynamic Formulation—A Critique of a Psychiatric Ritual," *American Journal of Psychiatry* 125(12):1738-1742, 1969.

14. K. M. Bowman and M. Rose, "A Criticism of the Terms 'Psychosis,' 'Psychoneurosis,' and 'Neurosis,'" *American Journal of Psychiatry* 108:161-166, 1951. See also: O. Diethelm, "The Fallacy of the Concept: Psychosis," in *Current Problems in Psychiatric Diagnosis*, eds., P. H. Hoch and J. Zubin (New York: Grune & Stratton, 1953) pp. 24-32.

15. D. L. Rosenhan, "On Being Sane in Insane Places," *Science* 179:250-258, January 19, 1973.

16. M. K. Temerlin and W. W. Trousdale, "The Social Psychology of Clinical Diagnosis," *Psychotherapy: Theory, Research and Practice* 6(1):24-29, 1969. See also: M. K. Temerlin, "Suggestion Effects in Psychiatric Diagnosis," *Journal of Nervous and Mental Disease* 147(4):349-353, 1968.

17. P. Ash, "The Reliability of Psychiatric Diagnoses," *Journal of Abnormal and Social Psychology* 44:272-276, 1949.

18. A. T. Beck et al., "Reliability of Psychiatric Diagnoses: 2. A Study of Consistency of Clinical Judgments and Ratings," *American Journal of Psychiatry* 119(4):351-357, 1962; H. O. Schmidt and C. P. Fanda, "The Reliability of Psychiatric Diagnosis, A New Look," *Journal of Abnormal and Social Psychology* 52(2):262-267, 1956; B. Mehlman, "The Reliability of Psychiatric Diagnoses," *Journal of Abnormal and Social Psychology* 47(2, supplement):577-578, 1952; and D. Conover, "Psychiatric Distinctions: New and Old Approaches," *Journal*

of Health and Social Behavior 13(2):167-180, 1972.

19. B. Pasamanick, S. Dinity, and M. Lefton, "Psychiatric Orientation and Its Relation to Diagnosis and Treatment in a Mental Hospital," *American Journal of Psychiatry* 116(2):127-132, 1959.

20. A. A. Rogow, *The Psychiatrists* (New York: Putnam's, 1970), p. 30. (Quoting S. A. Stauffler, *Measurement and Prediction; Studies in Social Psychology in World War II* (Princeton: Princeton University Press, 1950), pp. 473-477.)

21. H. S. Hughes, *Consciousness and Society: The Reorientation of European Social Thought 1890-1930* (New York: Knopf, 1958).

22. "Giveaway Man Flops with Nixon," *San Francisco Chronicle*, January 20, 1970, p. 3.

23. M. Jahoda, *Current Concepts of Positive Mental Health*, Joint Commission on Mental Illness and Health (New York: Basic Books, 1958), p. 73.

24. Ibid., p. 119.

25. M. Sabshin, "Psychiatric Perspectives on Normality," *Archives of General Psychiatry* 17(3):258-264, 1967.

26. E. H. Ackerknecht, "Psychopathology, Primitive Medicine, and Primitive Culture," *Bulletin of the History of Medicine* 14:30-67, 1943.

27. L. Srole et al., *Mental Health in the Metropolis: The Midtown Manhattan Study* (New York: McGraw-Hill, 1962), p. 230.

28. A. Leighton, discussion in *Transcultural Psychiatry*, eds., A. V. S. DeReuck and R. Porter (Boston: Little, Brown, 1965).

29. "Mental Health Study Concludes Two-Thirds of Westchester's 3 to 18-Year Olds Suffer Impairment," *New York Times*, June 28, 1970, p. 52.

30. G. Engel, "Is Grief a Disease?" *Psychosomatic Medicine* 23(1):18-22, 1961. See also: G. L. Engel, "Unified Concept of Health and Disease," *Perspective in Biology and Medicine* 3:459-485, 1960.

CHAPTER 5

1. A. A. Rogow, *The Psychiatrists* (New York: Putnam's, 1970).

2. W. E. Henry, J. H. Sims, and S. L. Spray, *The Fifth Profession* (San Francisco: Jossey-Bass, 1971). See also: A. S. Mariner, "A Critical Look at Professional Education in the Mental Health Field," *American Psychologist* 22:271-281, 1967.

3. H. Kaplan, "Should Psychiatrists Do Physical Examinations on Their Patients?" *Journal of the American Medical Association* 216(5):892, 1971.

4. T. S. Szasz, "Psychoanalysis and Taxation." *American Journal of Psychotherapy* 18:635-643, 1964.

5. G. W. Albee, "The Miracle of the Loaves and Fishes Updated: Non-Professionals for Everyone," in *Behavior Disorders: Perspectives and Trends,* ed., O. Milton (Philadelphia: Lippincott, 1973).

6. Ibid.

7. B. S. Brown and T. F. Courtless, "The Mentally Retarded in Penal and Correctional Institutions," *American Journal of Psychiatry* 124(9):1164-1170, 1968. See also: J. Fialka, "The Psychiatric Gap," *Washington Star,* January 17, 1972, pp. A-1 and A-8.

8. "Census of U.S. Psychiatric Manpower, 1971," mimeographed (Washington, D.C.: American Psychiatric Association). See also: E. F. Torrey, "Psychiatric Training: The SST of American Medicine," *Psychiatric Annals* 2(2):60-71, 1972.

9. W. Ryan, ed., *Distress in the City* (Cleveland: Press of Case Western Reserve University, 1969).

10. D. A. Hamburg, et al., "Report of Ad Hoc Committee on Central Fact-Gathering Data of the American Psychoanalytic Association," *Journal of the American Psychoanalytic Association* 15:841-861, 1967.

11. W. Weintraub and H. Aronson, "Is Classical Psychoanalysis a Dangerous Procedure?" *Journal of Nervous and Mental Disease* 149:224-228, 1969.

12. F. C. Redlich and D. X. Freedman, *The Theory and Practice of Psychiatry* (New York: Basic Books, 1966), p. 270.

13. S. K. Pande, "The Mystique of 'Western' Psychotherapy: An Eastern Interpretation," *Journal of Nervous and Mental Disease* 146(6):425-432, 1968. See also: V. D. Sauna, "Socio-Cultural Aspects of Psychotherapy and Treatment: A Review of the Literature," in *Progress in Clinical Psychology* (New York: Grune & Stratton, 1966).

14. B. Kaplan and D. Johnson, "The Social Meaning of Navaho Psychopathology and Psychotherapy," in *Magic, Faith, and Healing,* ed., A. Kiev (New York: The Free Press, 1964).

15. S. Nishimaru, "Mental Climate and Eastern Psychotherapy," *Transcultural Psychiatric Research* 2:24, April 1965.

16. K. Davis, "Mental Hygiene and the Class Structure," *Psychiatry* 1:55-65, 1938.

17. O. R. Gursslin, R. G. Hunt, and J. L. Roach, "Social Class and the Mental Health Movement," in *Mental Health of the Poor,* eds., F. Riessman, J. Cohen, and A. Pearl (New York:'The Free Press, 1964). See also: B. Wootton, *Social Science and Social Pathology* (London: George Allen and Unwin, 1959).

18. E. G. Poser, "The Effect of Therapists' Training on Group Therapeutic Outcome," *Journal of Consulting Psychology* 30(4):283-289, 1966.

19. G. O. Ebersole, P. H. Liederman, and I. D. Yalom, "Training the Non-Professional Group Therapist," *Journal of Nervous and Mental Disease* 149(3):294-302, 1969.

20. E. F. Torrey, *The Mind Game: Witchdoctors and Psychiatrists* (New York: Emerson, 1972). See also: E. F. Torrey, "The Case for the Indigenous Therapist," *Archives of General Psychiatry* 20:365-373, 1969.

21. Ibid.

22. C. M. Pierce, J. L. Mathis, and V. Pishkin, "Basic Psychiatry in Twelve Hours," *Diseases of the Nervous System* 29:533-535, 1968.

23. M. P. Dumont, *The Absurd Healer: Perspectives of a Community Psychiatrist* (New York: Science House, 1968). Dumont agrees that all other arguments are absurd.

24. E. Goffman, *Asylums: Essays on the Social Situation of Mental Patients and Other Inmates* (Garden City, N.Y.: Anchor Books, 1961).

25. R. Maisel, "Decision-Making in a Commitment Court," *Psychiatry* 33(3):352-361, 1970.

26. Ibid.

27. T. S. Szasz, *The Manufacture of Mad-*

ness: A Comparative Study of the Inquisition and the Mental Health Movement (New York: Dell, 1970), p. 65.

28. B. J. Ennis, *Prisoners of Psychiatry: Mental Patients, Psychiatrists and the Law* (New York: Harcourt Brace Jovanovich, 1972), p. 215. Also personal communication, Office of Information, Bureau of Prisons, United States Department of Justice.

29. "Preliminary Findings for the Psychiatric Inventory of Saint Elizabeth's Hospital," mimeographed (Washington, D.C.: Prepared by the Hospital Staff, May 31, 1970).

30. Personal communication, Associate Warden for Custody, Leavenworth Federal Prison, May 1971.

31. K. Kesey, *One Flew Over the Cuckoo's Nest* (New York: Viking, 1962). For an example of a prisoner who learned the rule, see: P. A. McCombs, "Free After 6 Years of Silence," *Washington Post*, June 22, 1972, pp. B1 and B4.

32. "Mental Patients' Rights," *Civil Liberties*, pp. 3-6, September 1972.

33. N. N. Kittrie, *The Right To Be Different: Deviance and Enforced Therapy* (Baltimore: Johns Hopkins Press, 1971), p. 98.

34. G. Bliss and P. Zekman, "Blunders Helped Advance Imposter," *Chicago Tribune*, March 1, 1972, p. 1.

35. P. Zekman and G. Bliss, "Ogilvie Plans Tighter Reins on State's Unlicensed Medics," *Chicago Tribune*, March 5, 1972, p. 2.

36. For more on this problem, see: E. F. Torrey, "Cheap Labor from Poor Nations," *American Journal of Psychiatry* 130(4):428-433, 1973.

37. P. R. Breggin, "The Return of Psychosurgery: An Analysis and Review," mimeographed (Washington School of Psychiatry, 1972).

38. J. M. R. Delgado, *Physical Control of the Mind: Toward a Psychocivilized Society* (New York: Harper and Row, 1969), pp. 200, 220, and 258.

39. L. H. Cotter, "Operant Conditioning in a Vietnamese Mental Hospital," *American Journal of Psychiatry* 124(1):23-28, 1967.

40. G. W. Albee, "Myths, Models, and Manpower," *Mental Hygiene* 52(2):168-180, 1968. See also: Albee, "The Miracle of the Loaves and Fishes Updated." See also: Kittrie,

The Right To Be Different: Deviance and Enforced Therapy.

41. B. M. Braginsky, D. D. Braginsky, and K. Ring, *Methods of Madness: The Mental Hospital as a Last Resort* (New York: Holt, Rinehart and Winston, 1969).

42. Ibid., p. 162. A study of inmates of an institution for the "mentally retarded" which makes this same point is: R. B. Edgerton and H. F. Dingman, "Good Reasons for Bad Supervision: 'Dating' in a Hospital for the Mentally Retarded," *Psychiatric Quarterly Supplement* 38:221-233, 1964.

43. J. E. Rappeport and G. Lassen, "Dangerousness—Arrest Rate Comparison of Discharged Patients and the General Population," *American Journal of Psychiatry* 121:776-783, 1965.

44. Ibid.

45. L. H. Cohen and H. Freeman, "How Dangerous to the Community Are State Hospital Patients?" *Connecticut State Medical Journal* 9:697-700, 1945. For further evidence, see also: J. R. Rappeport, *The Clinical Evaluation of the Dangerousness of the Mentally Ill* (Springfield, Ill.: Charles C. Thomas, 1967).

46. H. J. Steadman, "The Psychiatrist as a Conservative Agent of Social Control," *Social Problems* 20(2):263-271, 1972. See also: H. J. Steadman, "Follow-up on Baxstrom Patients Returned to Hospitals for the Criminally Insane," *American Journal of Psychiatry* 130(3):317-319, 1973.

47. Szasz, *The Manufacture of Madness*, p. XXVII. See also the epilogue of the book, which is relevant.

48. W. M. Mendel, "On the Abolition of the Psychiatric Hospital," in *Comprehensive Mental Health*, eds., C. M. Roberts, N. S. Greenfield, and M. H. Miller (Madison: University of Wisconsin Press, 1968).

49. Ibid.

50. P. W. Valentine, "Most at St. Elizabeth's Called Well Enough to Leave," *Washington Post*, August 11, 1971.

51. Mendel, "On the Abolition of the Psychiatric Hospital."

CHAPTER 6

1. J. C. Nunnally, *Popular Conceptions of Mental Health* (New York: Holt,

Rinehart and Winston, 1961). See also: B. J. Ennis, *Prisoners of Psychiatry: Mental Patients, Psychiatrists and the Law* (New York: Harcourt Brace Jovanovich, 1972).

2. E. Crumpton et al., "How Patients and Normals See the Mental Patient," *Journal of Clinical Psychology* 23:46-49, 1967; W. J. Johannsen, "Attitudes Toward Mental Patients: A Review of Empirical Research," *Mental Hygiene* 53(2):218-228, 1969; O. H. Mowrer, "Sin, the Lesser of Two Evils," *American Psychologist* 15:301-304, 1960; and J. G. Rabkin, "Opinions About Mental Illness: A Review of the Literature," *Psychological Bulletin* 77(3):153-171, 1972.

3. A. Ellis, "Should Some People Be Labeled Mentally Ill?" *Journal of Consulting Psychology* 31(5):435-446, 1967.

4. T. R. Sarbin, "On the Futility of the Proposition that Some People be Labeled 'Mentally Ill'," *Journal of Consulting Psychology* 31:447-453, 1967.

5. A. Schweitzer, *The Psychiatric Study of Jesus* (Boston: Beacon Press, 1948).

6. T. S. Szasz, *Law, Liberty, and Psychiatry* (New York: Macmillan, 1963). p. 228.

7. T. S. Szasz, *Psychiatric Justice* (New York: Macmillan, 1965), p. 224.

8. Ibid.

9. R. Coles, "A Fashionable Kind of Slander," *Atlantic Monthly*, November 1970.

10. M. M. Klein and S. A. Grossman, "Voting Competence and Mental Health," *American Journal of Psychiatry* 127(11):1562-1565, 1971.

11. R. J. Simon, "Mental Patients as Jurors," *Human Organization* 22(4):276-282, Winter 1963-1964.

12. H. Feifel, "Attitudes Toward Death in Some Normal and Mentally Ill Population," in *The Meaning of Death*, ed., H. Feifel (New York: McGraw-Hill, 1959), p. 117.

13. P. D. Lipsitt, D. Lelos, and A. L. McGarry, "Competency for Trial: A Screening Instrument," *American Journal of Psychiatry* 128(1):105-109, 1971. The 1972 Supreme Court decision Jackson versus Indiana will make this more difficult. Defendants who are found incompetent to stand trial will now also have to meet the standards required for involuntary

civil commitment. See also: National Institute of Mental Health, *Competency to Stand Trial and Mental Illness*, DHEW Publication No. 73-9105 (Washington, D.C.: Government Printing Office, 1973).

14. Ennis, *Prisoners of Psychiatry: Mental Patients, Psychiatrists and the Law*, p. 46.

15. Szasz, *Psychiatric Justice*. See also: R. Barton and J. A. Whitehead, "The Gas-Light Phenomenon," *Lancet* 1:1258-1260, June 21, 1969.

16. "Incompetency Commitments Held Excessive by Harvard Study," *Psychiatric News*, May 2, 1973, pp. 20-21. See also: *Competency to Stand Trial and Mental Illness*; and G. Cooke, N. Johnston, and E. Pogany, "Factors Affecting Referral to Determine Competency to Stand Trial," *American Journal of Psychiatry* 130(8):870-875, 1973.

17. Ibid.; and M. F. Abramson, "The Criminalization of Mentally Disordered Behavior: Possible Side-Effect of a New Mental Health Law," *Hospital and Community Psychiatry* 23:101-105, 1972.

18. Ibid.

19. "Macing Mental Patients," *Medical World News*, March 6, 1970, pp. 18-19.

20. Szasz, *Law, Liberty, and Psychiatry*, p. 249. For an analysis of the faulty logic behind this procedure, see also: J. M. Livermore, C. P. Malmquist, and P. E. Meehl, "On the Justifications for Civil Commitment," *University of Pennsylvania Law Review* 117:75-96, 1968.

21. T. J. Scheff, "The Societal Reaction to Deviance: Ascriptive Elements on the Psychiatric Screening of Mental Patients in a Midwestern State," *Social Problems* 11:401-413, 1964.

22. F. Cohen, "The Function of the Attorney and the Commitment of the Mentally Ill," *Texas Law Review* 44:424-469, 1966.

23. D. Miller and M. Schwartz, "County Lunacy Commission Hearings: Some Observations of Commitments to a State Mental Hospital," *Social Problems* 14:26-35, 1966.

24. R. Maisel, "Decision-Making in a Commitment Court," *Psychiatry* 33(3):352-361, 1970.

25. I. Solzhenitsyn, *One Day in the Life of Ivan Denisovich* (New York: Praeger, 1963).

26. Maisel. "Decision-Making in a Commitment Court." And to make matters worse, the "medical" testimony given is often of distinctly limited value. For instance, it has been shown that laymen are better predictors of dangerous behavior than the staff of a mental "hospital." See also: J. R. Rappeport, *The Clinical Evaluation of the Dangerousness of the Mentally Ill* (Springfield. Ill.: Charles C. Thomas, 1967).

27. Cohen. "The Function of the Attorney and the Commitment of the Mentally Ill."

28. "Freed After 59 Years." *New York Times*, May 1, 1964, p. 71.

29. "Forgotten Suspect 38 Years Later." *San Francisco Chronicle*, February 10, 1969.

30. Ennis. *Prisoners of Psychiatry: Mental Patients, Psychiatrists and the Law.*

31. *Mental Health Digest* 1(10):56-57, 1969. Quoting in re Sealy, 218 So. 2nd 765. District Court of Appeal of Florida. First District, February 13, 1969.

32. Szasz, *Law, Liberty, and Psychiatry.*

33. G. V. Morozov and I. M. Kalashnik, eds., *Forensic Psychiatry* (White Plains, N.Y.: International Arts & Sciences Press, 1970). Originally published in Russian in 1967, translated by M. Vale.

34. Ibid., p. 171.

35. Ibid., p. 168.

36. Ibid., p. 225.

37. A. S. Goldstein, *The Insanity Defense* (New Haven: Yale University Press, 1967), p. 3.

38. For a good description of this, see: S. Halleck, *Psychiatry and the Dilemmas of Crime* (New York: Harper and Row, 1967).

39. B. Wootton, *Social Science and Social Pathology* (London: George Allen and Unwin, 1959), p. 203.

40. For a more detailed analysis of this, see: S. Nelson and F. Torrey, "The Religious Functions of Psychiatry," *American Journal of Orthopsychiatry* 43(3):362-367, 1973.

41. A. M. Platt and B. L. Diamond, "The Origins and Development of the 'Wild Beast' Concept of Mental Illness and its Relations to Theories of Criminal Responsibility," *Journal of the History of the Behavioral Sciences* 1(4):355-367, 1965.

42. G. Zilboorg and G. W. Henry, *A History of Medical Psychology* (New York: Norton, 1941), p. 239.

43. Some observers contended that the Durham Rule, despite its original intentions, turned out to be less liberal than the McNaughton Rule. See: R. Arens, *Make Mad the Guilty. The Insanity Defense in the District of Columbia* (Springfield, Ill.: Charles C. Thomas, 1969).

44. J. Mann, "Defendants Restricted on Insanity Plea," *Washington Post*, June 24, 1972, pp. 1 and 10.

45. D. L. Bazelon, "Psychiatry's Fear of Analysis." *Washington Post*, June 24, 1973.

46. Szasz, *Psychiatric Justice*, p. 53.

47. Accounts of the trial are from the *New York Times* and the *San Francisco Chronicle*, March and April 1969.

48. G. Wright, "Sirhan's Psyche Show," *San Francisco Examiner and Chronicle*, April 20, 1969.

49. "The Psychiatric Mess in Court," *San Francisco Chronicle*, August 27, 1968.

50. R. Lindsey, "Sane or Insane? A Case Study of the TWA Hijacker," *New York Times*, January 18, 1973, pp. 43 and 49.

51. Goldstein, *The Insanity Defense*, p. 221.

52. "Modern Legal Test on Insanity Attacked by One of Its Drafters," *New York Times*, August 30, 1970.

53. K. Menninger, *The Crime of Punishment* (New York: Viking Press, 1966).

54. S. L. Halleck and W. Bromberg, *Psychiatric Aspects of Criminology* (Springfield, Ill.: Charles C. Thomas, 1968).

55. J. P. MacKenzie, "Nixon Details Anti-Crime Law Package," *Washington Post*, March 15, 1973, pp. 1 and 12.

CHAPTER 7

1. H. J. Leuchter, "Are Schools To Be or Not To Be Mental Health Centers?" *American Journal of Psychiatry* 125(4):575-576, 1968.

2. G. Rosen, *Madness in Society: Chapters in the Historical Sociology of Mental Illness* (New York: Harper and Row, 1968).

3. G. Caplan and H. Grunebaum, "Perspectives on Primary Prevention," *Archives of General Psychiatry* 17:331-346, 1967.

4. R. A. Schwartz, "The Role of Family Planning in the Primary Prevention of

Mental Illness," *American Journal of Psychiatry* 125(12):1711-1718, 1969.

5. C. Rhead et al., "The Psychological Assessment of Police Candidates," *American Journal of Psychiatry* 124(11):1575-1580, 1968.

6. J. O'Connell, "The Crazy Driver, the Car Maker, and Psychiatry. Letters to the Editor," *American Journal of Psychiatry* 124(8):1140-1142, 1968.

7. Caplan and Grunebaum, "Perspectives on Primary Prevention."

8. Committee on Social Issues, *The Social Responsibility of Psychiatrists: A Statement of Orientation* (New York: Group for the Advancement of Psychiatry, 1950).

9. The Committee on Social Issues. *Considerations Regarding the Loyalty Oath as a Manifestation of Current Social Tension and Anxiety* (New York: Group for the Advancement of Psychiatry, 1954).

10. Group for the Advancement of Psychiatry. *The Dimensions of Community Psychiatry* (New York: Group for the Advancement of Psychiatry, 1968).

11. H. M. Freed, "The Community Psychiatrist and Political Action," *Archives of General Psychiatry* 17:129-134, 1967. See also: W. Ryan, ed., *Distress in the City* (Cleveland: Press of Case Western Reserve University, 1969).

12. A. Macleod and P. Poland, "The Well-Being Clinic," *Social Work*, pp. 13-18, 1961.

13. F. Fanon, *Black Skin, White Masks* (New York: Grove Press, 1967).

14. F. Fanon, *The Wretched of the Earth* (New York: Grove Press, 1966).

15. F. Fanon, *A Dying Colonialism* (Middlesex, England: Penguin Books, 1959).

16. Fanon, *Black Skin, White Masks.*

17. P. L. Adams, "The Social Psychiatry of Frantz Fanon," *American Journal of Psychiatry* 127(6):809-814, 1970.

18. D. Caute, *Frantz Fanon* (New York: Viking Press, 1970).

19. I. L. Gendzier, *Frantz Fanon: A Critical Study* (New York: Pantheon, 1973).

20. N. V. Lourie and D. Walden, "The Lessons of Historical Reform Movements—the Racism-Mental Health Equation," *American Journal of Orthopsychiatry*, 40(4):251, 1970.

21. L. J. Duhl, ed., *The Urban Condition: People and Policy in the Metropolis* (New York: Basic Books, 1963). L. J. Duhl and R. L. Leopold, eds., *Mental Health and Urban Social Policy: A Casebook of Community Actions* (San Francisco: Jossey-Bass, 1968).

22. L. J. Duhl, "The Shame of the Cities," *American Journal of Psychiatry* 124(9):1184-1189, 1968.

23. R. Coles, *Children of Crisis* (Boston: Little, Brown, 1964).

24. R. Coles and H. Huge, "Strom Thurmond Country: The Way It Is in South Carolina," *New Republic*, pp. 17-21, November 30, 1968.

25. "Feeding the Hungry," *New Republic*, p. 11, March 15, 1969.

26. R. Coles, *Children of Crisis*, p. 381.

27. B. L. Bloom, "The Evaluation of Primary Prevention Programs," in *Comprehensive Mental Health*, eds., L. M. Roberts, N. S. Greenfield, and M. H. Miller (Madison: University of Wisconsin Press, 1968).

28. B. L. Bloom, "The 'Medical Model', Miasma Theory, and Community Mental Health," *Community Mental Health Journal* 1:333-338, 1965.

29. W. G. Burrows, "Community Psychiatry—Another Bandwagon?" *Canadian Psychiatric Association Journal* 14:105-114, 1969.

30. J. S. Bockoven, "Community Psychiatry: A Growing Source of Social Confusion," *Psychiatry Digest* pp. 51-60, 1968.

31. F. C. Redlich and M. Pepper, "Are Social Psychiatry and Community Psychiatry Subspecialities of Psychiatry?" *American Journal of Psychiatry* 124(10):1343-1350, 1968.

32. T. S. Szasz, *Law, Liberty, and Psychiatry* (New York: Macmillan, 1963).

33. R. Leifer, *In the Name of Mental Health: The Social Functions of Psychiatry* (New York: Science House, 1969).

34. H. W. Dunham, "Community Psychiatry: The Newest Therapeutic Bandwagon," *Archives of General Psychiatry* 12:303-313, 1965.

35. D. L. Bazelon, "Follow the Yellow Brick Road," *American Journal of Orthopsychiatry* 40(4):562-567, 1970.

36. "Smut Pouring into City," *San Francisco Chronicle*, December 18, 1969.

37. S. Nelson and F. Torrey, "The Religious Functions of Psychiatry," *American Journal of Orthopsychiatry* 43(3):362-367, 1973.

38. L. S. Kubie, "Commitment," *Psychiatry News* March 21, 1973, p. 2.

39. B. Wootton, *Social Science and Social*

Pathology (London: George Allen and Unwin, 1959). See also: "Outpatient Therapy Ordered," *Washington Post*, April 30, 1972.

40. "Psychiatrists Oppose Registries," *Journal of the American Medical Association* 214(6):1128, 1970.

41. G. B. Chisholm, "The Reestablishment of Peacetime Society: The Responsibility of Psychiatry," *Psychiatry* 9:3-11, 1946.

42. L. K. Frank, *Society as the Patient* (New Brunswick: Rutgers University Press, 1948). p. 1.

43. Ibid., p. 156.

44. L. Bellak, "Toward Control of Today's Epidemic of Mental Disease," *Medical World News*, February 6, 1970.

45. Ibid.

46. C. McCabe, "On Looney Leaders," *San Francisco Chronicle*, September 30, 1969.

47. Bockoven, "Community Psychiatry."

48. K. Keniston, "How Community Mental Health Stamped Out the Riots (1968-78)," *Transaction* 5(8):21-29, 1968.

49. Ryan, *Distress in the City*.

CHAPTER 8

1. N. Postman and C. Weingartner, *Teaching as a Subversive Activity* (New York: Delacorte, 1969).

2. C. E. Silberman, *Crisis in the Classroom* (New York: Random House, 1970).

3. Postman and Weingartner, *Teaching as a Subversive Activity*.

CHAPTER 9

1. C. R. Rogers, "The Increasing Involvement of the Psychologist in Social Problems: Some Comments, Positive and Negative," *Journal of Applied Behavioral Science* 5(1):3, 1969.

2. *American Anthropologist* 72:6, 1970.

3. R. Dubos, *Man Adapting* (New Haven: Yale University Press, 1965).

4. R. Ekstein and R. L. Motto, "Psychoanalyses and Education: A Reappraisal," *Psychoanalytic Review* 51(4):29-44, 1964-1965.

5. A. S. Neill, *Summerhill* (New York: Hart, 1960).

6. W. Allinsmith and G. W. Goethals, *The Role of Schools in Mental Health*,

Monograph Series No. 7, Joint Commission on Mental Illness and Health (New York: Basic Books, 1962).

7. D. Rogers, *Mental Hygiene in Elementary Education* (Boston: Houghton Mifflin, 1957), p. 185.

8. L. S. Kubie, "The Psychotherapeutic Ingredient in the Learning Process," in *The Role of Learning in Psychotherapy*, ed., R. Porter (Boston: Little, Brown, 1968).

9. T. S. Szasz, *The Ethics of Psychoanalysis* (New York: Basic Books, 1965). See also: T. S. Szasz, "Whither Psychiatry?" *Social Research* 33(3):439-462, 1966.

10. J. Wilson, *Education and the Concept of Mental Health* (London: Routledge and Kegan Paul, 1969).

11. R. M. Jones, *Fantasy and Feeling in Education* (New York: New York University Press, 1968).

12. H. C. Lyon, *Learning to Feel—Feeling to Learn* (Columbus: Merrill, 1971).

13. G. I. Brown, *Human Teaching for Human Learning* (New York: Viking Press, 1971).

14. See, for example: G. Weinstein and M. D. Fantin, *Toward Humanistic Education: A Curriculum of Affect* (New York: Praeger, 1970).

15. Committee on Preventive Psychiatry, *Promotion of Mental Hygiene in the Primary and Secondary Schools: An Evaluation of Four Projects*, Group for the Advancement of Psychiatry, 1951.

16. J. R. Seeley, *The Americanization of the Unconscious* (New York: International Science Press, 1967).

17. S. R. Roen, "Primary Prevention in the Classroom Through a Teaching Program in the Behavioral Sciences," in *Emergent Approaches to Mental Health Problems*, eds., E. L. Cowan, E. A. Gardner, and M. Zax (New York: Appleton-Century-Crofts, 1967). See also: S. R. Roen, "The Behavioral Sciences in the Primary Grades," *American Psychologist* 20:430-432, 1965.

18. Brown, *Human Teaching for Human Learning*.

19. Committee on Preventive Psychiatry, *Promotion of Mental Hygiene in the Primary and Secondary Schools*, p. 12. See also: R. H. Ojemann, "Investigation on the Effects of Teaching an Understanding and Appreciation of Behavior Dynamics," in *Prevention of Mental Disorders in Children*, ed., G.

Caplan (New York: Basic Books, 1961), pp. 378-397.

20. *People Watching* (New York: Behavioral Publications).

21. C. R. Rogers, *On Becoming a Person: A Therapist's View of Psychotherapy* (Boston: Houghton Mifflin, 1961), p. 276.

22. Ibid., p. 280. See also: C. R. Rogers, "The Interpersonal Relationship in the Facilitation of Learning," in *The Helping Relationship Sourcebook*, eds., D. L. Avila, A. W. Combs, and W. W. Purkey (Boston: Allyn & Bacon, 1971).

23. C. B. Truax and R. R. Carkhuff, *Toward Effective Counseling and Psychotherapy: Training and Practice* (Chicago: Aldine Publishing, 1967).

24. B. M. Brown, "Cognitive Aspects of Wolpe's Behavior Therapy," *American Journal of Psychiatry* 124(6):854-859, 1967.

25. C. R. Rogers, *Client-Centered Therapy* (Boston: Houghton Mifflin, 1951), p. 384.

26. Rogers, "The Interpersonal Relationship in the Facilitation of Learning," pp. 226-227.

27. D. N. Aspy, "A Study of Three Facilitative Conditions and Their Relationships to the Achievement of Third Grade Students" (Ph.D. diss., University of Kentucky, 1965. For summary, see: Truax and Carkhuff, *Toward Effective Counseling and Psychotherapy: Training and Practice.)*

28. D. N. Aspy, "Reaction to Carkhuff's Articles," *The Counseling Psychologist* 3(3):35-41, 1972.

29. D. N. Aspy, *Toward a Technology for Humanizing Education* (Champaign, Ill.: Research Press, 1972).

30. D. W. Soper and A. W. Combs, "The Helping Relationship as Seen by Teachers and Therapists," *Journal of Consulting Psychology* 26:288, 1962. See also: F. E. Fiedler, "Quantitative Studies on the Role of Therapists' Feelings Toward Their Patients" in *Psychotherapy: Theory and Research*, ed., O. H. Mowrer (New York: Ronald Press, 1953).

31. A. W. Combs, D. L. Avila, and W. W. Purkey, *Helping Relationships: Basic Concepts for the Helping Professions* (Boston: Allyn & Bacon, 1971), p. 10.

32. Rogers, "The Interpersonal Relationship in the Facilitation of Learning," p. 228.

33. C. E. Moustakas, *The Authentic Teacher: Sensitivity and Awareness in the Classroom* (Cambridge, Mass.: Doyle, 1966), p. 14.

34. W. Glasser, *Schools Without Failure* (New York: Harper and Row, 1969).

35. Lyon, *Learning to Feel—Feeling to Learn*, pp. 8-9 for a review of some of these. See also: Combs, Avila, and Purkey, *Helping Relationships: Basic Concepts for the Helping Professions;* R. Rosenthal and L. Jacobson, *Pygmalion in The Classroom* (New York: Holt, Rinehart and Winston, 1968); and R. Rosenthal, "The Pygmalion Effect Lives," *Psychology Today* 7(4):56-63, 1973.

36. A. Stunkard, "Some Interpersonal Aspects of an Oriental Religion," *Psychiatry* 14:419-431, 1951; N. W. Ross, *Three Ways of Asian Wisdom* (New York: Simon & Schuster, 1966); D. M. Burns, *Buddhist Meditation and Depth Psychology* (Kandy, Ceylon: Buddhist Publication Society, 1966); A. W. Watts, *Psychotherapy East and West* (New York: Pantheon, 1961); and E. F. Torrey, "Observations on Buddhism and Psychiatry in Thailand," *World Fellowship of Buddhists Bulletin* 7(1):16-19, 1970.

37. Combs, Avila, and Purkey, *Helping Relationships: Basic Concepts for the Helping Professions*, p. 4.

CHAPTER 10

1. C. S. Ford and F. A. Beach, *Patterns of Sexual Behavior* (New York: Harper and Row, 1951). See also: J. Marmor, " 'Normal' and 'Deviant' Sexual Behavior," *Journal of the American Medical Association* 217(2):165-170, 1971; and R. Green, "Homosexuality as a Mental Illness," *International Journal of Psychiatry* 10(1):77-98, 1972.

2. P. Solomon, "The Burden of Responsibility in Suicide and Homicide," *Journal of the American Medical Association* 199:321-324, 1967.

3. J. A. M. Meerloo, "Hidden Suicide," in *Suicidal Behaviors*, ed., H. L. P. Resnik (Boston: Little, Brown, 1968).

4. T. S. Szasz, *The Manufacture of Madness: A Comparative Study of the Inquisition and the Mental Health Movement* (New York: Dell, 1970).

5. C. MacAndrew, "On the Notion that Certain Persons Who Are Given to Frequent Drunkenness Suffer from a Disease called Alcoholism," in *Changing Perspectives in Mental Illness*, eds., S. C. Plog and R. B. Edgerton (New York: Holt, Rinehart and Winston, 1969).

6. S. C. McMorris, "Can We Punish for the Acts of Addiction?" *Bulletin on Narcotics* 22(3):43-48, 1970.

7. N. N. Kittrie, *The Right To Be Different: Deviance and Enforced Therapy* (Baltimore: Johns Hopkins Press, 1971).

8. W. Ryan, ed., *Distress in the City* (Cleveland: Press of Case Western Reserve University, 1969). See also: D. A. Hamburg et al., "Report of Ad Hoc Committee on Central Fact-Gathering Data of the American Psychoanalytic Association," *Journal of the American Psychoanalytic Association* 15:841-861, 1967.

9. G. J. Tucker et al., "The Relationship of Subtle Neurological Impairments to Disturbances of Thinking." Read before the Second Congress of International College of Psychosomatic Medicine, Amsterdam, 1973.

10. K. Davison and C. R. Bagley, "Schizophrenia-like Psychosis Associated with Organic Disorders of the Central Nervous System: A Review of the Literature," in *Current Problems in Neuropsychiatry*, ed., R. N. Herrington Special Publication No. 4 of *British Journal of Psychiatry*, Ashford, England: Headley Bros., 1969.

11. W. J. Fessel, "Blood Proteins in Functional Psychosis," *Archives of General Psychiatry* 6:40-56, 1962.

12. H. Y. Meltzer, "Creatine Phosphokinase Activity and Clinical Symptomatology," *Archives of General Psychiatry* 29:589-593, 1973.

13. E. F. Torrey and M. R. Peterson, "Slow and Latent Viruses in Schizophrenia," *Lancet* 2:22-24, July 7, 1973.

14. D. Hawkins and L. Pauling, eds., *Orthomolecular Psychiatry* (San Francisco: Freeman, 1973).

15. R. R. Fieve, J. Mendlewicz, and J. L. Fleiss, "Manic-Depressive Illness: Linkage with the Xg Blood Group," *American Journal of Psychiatry* 130(12):1355-1359, 1973.

16. R. D. Laing, *The Politics of Experience* (New York: Pantheon Books, 1967), p. 58.

CHAPTER 11

1. "Braceland Chides Law School Dean on Commitment Issue." *Psychiatric News*, May 2, 1973, p. 19. For the story of a young woman who would probably still be alive if voluntary retreats were available, see: P. Hodge, "A Disturbed Life and a Violent Death," *Washington Post*, February 14, 1973, p. 1. She wanted help but she refused to define herself as sick.

2. M. T. Kaufman, "Camp Offers a Haven for 1,000 of Bowery's Homeless," *New York Times*, December 18, 1972.

3. M. Satchell, "Retarded Are Easy Prey," *Washington Star-News*, August 7, 1973, p. 1.

4. M. Jones, *The Therapeutic Community* (New York: Basic Books, 1953).

5. B. M. Braginsky, D. C. Braginsky, and K. Ring, *Methods of Madness: The Mental Hospital as a Last Resort* (New York: Holt, Rinehart and Winston, 1969). See also: A. Toffler, *Future Shock* (New York: Random House, 1970), pp. 390-392.

6. K. I. Pearce, "A Comparison of Care Given by Family Practitioners and Psychiatrists in a Teaching Hospital Psychiatric Unit," *American Journal of Psychiatry* 127(6):835-840, 1970.

7. D. M. McNair, D. M. Callahan, and M. Lorr, "Therapist 'Type' and Patient Response to Psychotherapy," *Journal of Consulting Psychology* 26:425-429, 1962.

8. C. R. Rogers, *Client-Centered Therapy* (Boston: Houghton Mifflin, 1951), p. 424.

9. R. Moore, "How Personality Difference of Students and Teachers Influence Students' Achievement," *People Watching* 2(1):31-34, 1972.

10. R. L. Taylor and E. F. Torrey, "The Pseudoregulation of American Psychiatry," *American Journal of Psychiatry* 129(6):658-662, 1972.

11. A. S. Mariner, "A Critical Look at Professional Education in the Mental Health Field," *American Psychologist* 22:271-281, 1967.

12. "Missouri Aims at Drug Assignment by Computer Setup," *Psychiatric News*, July 5, 1972.

CHAPTER 12

1. W. M. Mendel, "Responsibility in Health, Illness and Treatment," *Archives of General Psychiatry* 18:697-705, 1968.
2. National Institute of Mental Health, *Competency to Stand Trial and Mental Illness*, DHEW Publication No. 73-9105 (Washington, D.C.: Government Printing Office, 1973), p. 4.
3. T. S. Szasz, *Law, Liberty, and Psychiatry* (New York: Macmillan, 1963), p. 228.
4. A. M. Dershowitz, "Psychiatry in the Legal Process: A Knife that Cuts Both Ways," *Judicature* 51(10):370-377, 1968.
5. T. S. Szasz, "Whither Psychiatry?" *Social Research* 33(3):439-462, 1966. See also: T. S. Szasz, "Problems Facing Psychiatry: The Psychiatrist as Party to Conflict," in *Ethical Issues in Medicine: The Role of the Physician in Today's Society*, ed., E. F. Torrey (Boston: Little, Brown, 1968).
6. Dershowitz, "Psychiatry in the Legal Process."
7. J. Robitscher, "Courts, State Hospitals, and the Right to Treatment," *American Journal of Psychiatry* 129(3):298-304, 1972.
8. "Ex-Mental Patient: A Precedent-Setting Case," *Medical World News*, December 15, 1972, p. 54.
9. N. N. Kittrie, *The Right To Be Different: Deviance and Enforced Therapy* (Baltimore: Johns Hopkins Press, 1971), p. 347.

CHAPTER 13

1. S. A. Shah, "Community Mental Health and the Criminal Justice System: Some Issues and Problems," *Mental Hygiene* 54(1):1-12, 1970.

CHAPTER 14

1. T. S. Kuhn, *The Structure of Scientific Revolutions* (Chicago: University of Chicago Press, 1962).
2. F. J. Braceland, "The Relationship of Psychiatry to Medicine," *Psychiatry Digest* pp. 12-16, April 1969.
3. R. J. Arthur, "Social Psychiatry: An Overview," *American Journal of Psychiatry* 130(8):841-849, 1973.
4. J. R. Seeley, *The Americanization of the Unconscious* (New York: International Science Press, 1967).

Bibliography

Abdullah, S.; Jarvik, L. F.; Kato, T.; Johnston, W. C.; and Lanskrow, J. "Extra Y Chromosome and its Psychiatric Implications." *Archives of General Psychiatry* 21:497-501, 1969.

Abrams, G. M. "Setting Limits." *Archives of General Psychiatry* 19:113-119, 1968.

Abramson, M. F. "The Criminalization of Mentally Disordered Behavior: Possible Side-Effect of a New Mental Health Law." *Hospital and Community Psychiatry* 23:101-105, 1972.

Ackerknecht, E. H. "Psychopathology, Primitive Medicine, and Primitive Culture." *Bulletin of the History of Medicine* 14:30-67, 1943.

Adams, P. L. "The Social Psychiatry of Frantz Fanon." *American Journal of Psychiatry* 127(6):809-814, 1970.

Albee, G. W. "Emerging Concepts of Mental Illness and Models of Treatment: The Psychological Point of View." *American Journal of Psychiatry* 125(7):870-876, 1969.

———. "The Miracle of the Loaves and Fishes Updated: Non-Professionals for Everyone." In *Behavior Disorders: Perspectives and Trends,* edited by O. Milton. Philadelphia: Lippincott, 1973.

———. "Myths, Models, and Manpower." *Mental Hygiene* 52(2):168-180, 1968.

———. "A Spectre Is Haunting the Outpatient Clinic." In *Psychiatric Clinics in Transition,* edited by A. B. Tulipan, and S. Feldman. New York: Brunner/Mazel, 1969.

Alexander, F. G., and Selesnick, S. J. *The History of Psychiatry.* New York: Harper and Row, 1966.

Allinsmith, W., and Goethals, G. W. *The Role of Schools in Mental Health.* Monograph Series No. 7, Joint Commission on Mental Illness and Health. New York: Basic Books, 1962.

Alschuler, A. S. "Psychological Education." *Journal of Humanistic Psychology* 9(1):1-16, 1969.

Arens, R. *Make Mad the Guilty. The Insanity Defense in the District of Columbia.* Springfield, Ill.: Charles C. Thomas, 1969.

Arnhoff, F. N.; Rubenstein, E. A.; and Speisman, J. C. *Manpower for Mental Health.* Chicago: Aldine Publishing, 1969.

Arthur, R. J. "Social Psychiatry: An Overview." *American Journal of Psychiatry* 130(8):841-849, 1973.

Ash, P. "The Reliability of Psychiatric Diagnoses." *Journal of Abnormal and Social Psychology* 44:272-276, 1949.

Aspy, D. N. "Reaction to Carkhuff's Articles." *The Counseling Psychologist* 3(3):35-41, 1972.

———. "A Study of Three Facilitative Conditions and Their Relationships to the Achievement of Third Grade Students." Ph.D. dissertation, University of Kentucky, 1965. Summarized in: Truax, C. B., and Carkhuff, R. R. *Toward Effective Counseling and Psychotherapy: Training and Practice.* Chicago: Aldine Publishing, 1967.

———. *Toward A Technology for Humanizing Education.* Champaign, Ill.: Research Press, 1972.

Ausubel, D. P. "Personality Disorder in Disease." *American Psychologist* 16:69-74, 1961.

Baker, D. P. " 'Compulsive Workers' Viewed as Sick as Other Addicts." *Washington Post,* October 14, 1972, p. B-1.

Bandura, A. "Modelling Approaches to the Modification of Phobic Disorders." In *The Role of Learning in Psychotherapy,* edited by R. Porter. Boston: Little, Brown, 1968.

Barclay, J. R. "Franz Brentano and Sigmund Freud." *Journal of Existentialism* 5(17):1-36, 1964.

Barton, R., and Whitehead, J. A. "The Gas-Light Phenomenon." *Lancet* 1:1258-1260, June 21, 1969.

Basescu, S. "The Threat of Suicide in Psychotherapy." *American Journal of Psychotherapy* 19:99-105, 1965.

Bazelon, D. L. "Follow the Yellow Brick Road." *American Journal of Orthopsychiatry* 40(4):562-567, 1970.

———. "Psychiatry's Fear of Analysis." *Washington Post,* June 24, 1973.

Beck, A. T.; Ward, C. H.; Mendelson, M.; Mock, J. E.; and Erbaugh, J. K. "Reliability of Psychiatric Diagnoses: 2. A Study of Consistency of Clinical Judgements and Ratings." *American Journal of Psychiatry* 119(4):351-357, 1962.

Becker, E. *The Revolution in Psychiatry.* New York: The Free Press, 1964.

Bellak, L. "Toward Control of Today's Epidemic of Mental Disease." *Medical World News,* February 6, 1970.

Benedict, R. "Anthropology and the Abnormal." *Journal of General Psychology* 10:59-82, 1934.

Berne, E. *Games People Play: The Psychology of Human Relationships.* New York: Grove Press, 1964.

Bettis, M., and Roberts, R. E. "Mental Health Manpower." *Mental Hygiene* 53(2):163-175, 1969.

Bloom, B. L. "The Evaluation of Primary Prevention Programs." In *Comprehensive Mental Health,* edited by L. M. Roberts; N. S. Greenfield; and M. H. Miller. Madison: University of Wisconsin Press, 1968.

———. "The 'Medical Model,' Miasma Theory, and Community Mental Health." *Community Mental Health Journal* 1:333-338,1965.

Bockoven, J. S. "Community Psychiatry: A Growing Source of Social Confusion." *Psychiatry Digest,* pp. 51-60, 1968.

Bolman, W. M., and Westman, J. C. "Prevention of Mental Disorder—An Overview of Current Programs." *American Journal of Psychiatry* 123:1058-1068, 1967.

Bowman, K. M., and Rose, M. "A Criticism of the Terms 'Psychosis,' 'Psychoneurosis,' and 'Neurosis.' " *American Journal of Psychiatry* 108:161-166, 1951.

Braceland, F. J. "The Relationship of Psychiatry to Medicine." *Psychiatry Digest*, pp. 12-16, April 1969.

Braginsky, B. M.; Braginsky, D. D.; and Ring, K. *Methods of Madness: The Mental Hospital as a Last Resort.* New York: Holt, Rinehart and Winston, 1969.

Breggin, P. R. "The Return of Psychosurgery: An Analysis and Review." Washington School of Psychiatry, 1972, Mimeographed.

Brown, B. M. "Cognitive Aspects of Wolpe's Behavior Therapy." *American Journal of Psychiatry* 124(6):854-859, 1967.

Brown, B. S., and Courtless, T. F. "The Mentally Retarded in Penal and Correctional Institutions." *American Journal of Psychiatry* 124(9):1164-1170, 1968.

Brown, G. I. *Human Teaching for Human Learning.* New York: Viking Press, 1971.

Brown, M. "The New Body Psychotherapies." *Psychotherapy* 10(2):98-116, 1973.

Burns, D. M. *Buddhist Meditation and Depth Psychology.* Kandy, Ceylon: Buddhist Publication Society, 1966.

Burrows, W. G. "Community Psychiatry—Another Bandwagon?" *Canadian Psychiatric Association Journal* 14:105-114, 1969.

Calderone, M. S. "Pornography as a Public Health Problem." *American Journal of Public Health* 62(3):374-376, 1972.

Campbell, J. P., and Dunnette, M. D. "Effectiveness of T-Group Experiences in Managerial Training and Development." *Psychological Bulletin* 70(2):73-104, 1968.

Caplan, G., and Grunebaum, H. "Perspectives on Primary Prevention." *Archives of General Psychiatry* 17:331-346, 1967.

Caute, D. *Frantz Fanon.* New York: Viking Press, 1970.

Chisholm, G. B. "The Reestablishment of Peacetime Society: The Responsibility of Psychiatry." *Psychiatry* 9:3-11, 1946.

Cohen, F. "The Function of the Attorney and the Commitment of the Mentally Ill." *Texas Law Review* 44:424-469, 1966.

Cohen, L. H., and Freeman, H. "How Dangerous to the Community are State Hospital Patients?" *Connecticut State Medical Journal* 9:697-700, 1945.

Coles, R. *Children of Crisis.* Boston: Little, Brown & Co., 1964.

———. "A Fashionable Kind of Slander." *Atlantic Monthly,* November 1970.

———. "Observation or Participation: The Problem of Psychiatric Research on Social Issues." *Journal of Nervous and Mental Disease* 141(2):274-284, 1965.

——— and Huge, H. "Strom Thurmond Country: The Way It Is in South Carolina." *New Republic,* pp. 17-21, November 30, 1968.

Combs, A. W.; Avila, D. L.; and Purkey, W. W. *Helping Relationships: Basic Concepts for the Helping Professions.* Boston: Allyn & Bacon, 1971.

The Committee on Social Issues. *Considerations Regarding the Loyalty Oath as a Manifestation of Current Social Tension and Anxiety.* Symposium No. 1. New York: Group for the Advancement of Psychiatry, 1954.

Conover, D. "Psychiatric Distinctions: New and Old Approaches." *Journal of Health and Social Behavior* 13(2):167-180, 1972.

Cooke, G.; Johnston, N.; and Pogany, E. "Factors Affecting Referral to Determine Competency to Stand Trial." *American Journal of Psychiatry* 130(8):870-875, 1973.

Cotter, L. H. "Operant Conditioning in a Vietnamese Mental Hospital." *American Journal of Psychiatry* 124(1):23-28, 1967.

Crawshaw, R. "How Sensitive is Sensitivity Training?" *American Journal of Psychiatry* 126(6):868-873, 1969.

Crumpton, E.; Weinstein, A. D.; Acker, C. W.; and Annis, A. P. "How Patients and Normals See the Mental Patient." *Journal of Clinical Psychology* 23:46-49, 1967.

Daniels, D. N., and Kuldau, J. M. "Marginal Man, the Tether of Tradition, and Intentional Social Systems Therapy." *Community Mental Health Journal* 3(1):13-20, 1967.

Davis, K. "Mental Hygiene and the Class Structure." *Psychiatry* 1:55-65, 1938.

Davison, K., and Bagley, C. R. "Schizophrenia-like Psychosis Associated with Organic Disorder of the Central Nervous System: A Review of the Literature." In *Current Problems in Neuropsychiatry*, edited by R. N. Herrington. Special Publication No. 4 of *British Journal of Psychiatry*. Ashford, England: Headley Bros., 1969.

Delgado, J. M. R. *Physical Control of the Mind: Toward a Psychocivilized Society.* New York: Harper and Row, 1969.

deReuck, A. V. S., and Porter, R., eds. *The Mentally Abnormal Offender.* Ciba Foundation Symposium. Boston: Little, Brown, 1968.

Dershowitz, A. M. "Psychiatry in the Legal Process: A Knife that Cuts Both Ways." *Judicature* 51(10):370-377, 1968.

Diethelm, O. "The Fallacy of the Concept: Psychosis." In *Current Problems in Psychiatric Diagnosis*, edited by P. H. Hoch, and J. Zubin. New York: Grune & Stratton, 1953.

The Dimensions of Community Psychiatry. Report No. 69, New York: Group for the Advancement of Psychiatry, 1968.

Dreber, R. H. "Origin, Development and Present Status of Insanity as a Defense to Criminal Responsibility in the Common Law." *Journal of the History of the Behavioral Sciences* 3:47-57, 1967.

Dubos, R. *Man Adapting.* New Haven: Yale University Press, 1965.

Duhl, L. J. "The Shame of the Cities." *American Journal of Psychiatry* 124(9):1184-1189, 1969.

Duhl, L. J., ed. *Urban America and the Planning of Mental Health Services.* New York: Group for the Advancement of Psychiatry, 1964.

———. *The Urban Condition: People and Policy in the Metropolis.* New York: Basic Books, 1963.

——— and Leopold, R. L., eds. *Mental Health and Urban Social Policy: A Casebook of Community Actions.* San Francisco: Jossey-Bass, 1968.

Dumont, M. P. *The Absurd Healer: Perspectives of a Community Psychiatrist.* New York: Science House, 1968.

——— and Aldrich, C. K. "Family Care After a Thousand Years—A Crisis in the Tradition of St. Dymphna." *American Journal of Psychiatry* 119(2):116-121, August 1962.

Dunham, H. W. "Community Psychiatry: The Newest Therapeutic Bandwagon." *Archives of General Psychiatry* 12:303-313, 1965.

Ebersole, G. O.; Liederman, P. H.; and Yalom, I. D. "Training the Non-Professional Group Therapist." *Journal of Nervous and Mental Disease* 149(3):294-302, 1969.

Edgerton, R. B., and Dingman, H. F. "Good Reasons for Bad Supervision:

'Dating' in a Hospital for the Mentally Retarded." *Psychiatric Quarterly Supplement* 38:221-233, 1964.

Ekstein, R., and Motto, R. L. "Psychoanalysis and Education: A Reappraisal." *Psychoanalytic Review* 51(4):29-44, 1964-1965.

Ellis, A. "Rational-Emotive Psychotherapy." In *Counseling and Psychotherapy: An Overview*, edited by D. S. Arbuckle. New York: McGraw-Hill, 1967.

———. "Should Some People be Labeled Mentally Ill?" *Journal of Consulting Psychology* 31(5):435-446, 1967.

Engel, G. L. "Is Grief a Disease?" *Psychosomatic Medicine* 23(1):18-22, 1961.

———. "Unified Concept of Health and Disease." *Perspectives in Biology and Medicine* 3:459-485, 1960.

Ennis, B. J. *Prisoners of Psychiatry: Mental Patients, Psychiatrists and the Law*. New York: Harcourt Brace Jovanovich, 1972.

Fanon, F. *Black Skin, White Masks*. New York: Grove Press, 1967.

———. *A Dying Colonialism*. Middlesex, England: Penguin Books, 1959.

———. *The Wretched of the Earth*. New York: Grove Press, 1966.

Federal Bureau of Prisons Statistical Report, Fiscal Year 1967 and 1968. Washington, D.C.: U.S. Department of Justice, Bureau of Prisons, 1969.

Feifel, H. "Attitudes Toward Death in Some Normal and Mentally Ill Populations." In *The Meaning of Death*, edited by H. Feifel. New York: McGraw-Hill, 1959.

Felix, R. "Psychiatrist, Medicinae Doctor." *American Journal of Psychiatry* 118:1-9, 1961.

Fellner, C. H. "Paperback Psychiatry." *Journal of Medical Education* 44(7):585-588, 1969.

Fessel, W. J., Blood Proteins in Functional Psychosis. *Archives of General Psychiatry* 6, 40-56, 1962.

Fiedler, F. E. "Quantitative Studies on the Role of Therapists' Feelings Toward Their Patients." In *Psychotherapy: Theory and Research*, edited by O. H. Mowrer. New York: Ronald Press, 1953.

Field, F. *The Last Days of Mankind: Karl Kraus and His Vienna.* New York: St. Martin's Press, 1967.

Fieve, R. R.; Mendlewicz, J.; and Fleiss, J. L. "Manic-Depressive Illness: Linkage with the Xg Blood Group." *American Journal of Psychiatry* 130(12):1355-1359, 1973.

Finch, S. M. "Nomenclature for Children's Mental Disorders Need Improvement." *International Journal of Psychiatry* 7(6):415, 1969.

Ford, C. S., and Beach, F. A. *Patterns of Sexual Behavior*. New York: Harper and Row, 1951.

Foucault, M. *Madness and Civilization: A History of Insanity in the Age of Reason*. New York: Random House, 1965.

Fox, S. J. *Science and Justice: The Massachusetts Witchcraft Trials*. Baltimore: Johns Hopkins Press, 1968.

Frank, L. K. "Society as the Patient." *American Journal of Sociology* 42:335-344, 1936.

———. *Society as the Patient*. New Brunswick: Rutgers University Press, 1948.

Freed, H. M. "The Community Psychiatrist and Political Action." *Archives of General Psychiatry* 17:129-134, 1967.

Freeman, T. "The Learning Component in the Dynamic Psychotherapeutic Situation." In *The Role of Learning in Psychotherapy*, edited by R. Porter. Boston: Little, Brown, 1968.

Freud, S. *Autobiography*. New York: Norton, 1935.

―――. "Postscript to a Discussion on Lay Analysts (1927)." In *The History of the Psychoanalytic Movement*. New York: Collier Books, 1963.

Friedes, D. "Toward the Elimination of the Concept of Normality." *Journal of Consulting Psychology* 24:128-133, 1960.

Fromm, E. *The Crisis of Psychoanalysis*. New York: Holt, Rinehart and Winston, 1970.

Galdston, I., ed. *Historic Derivations of Modern Psychiatry*. New York: McGraw-Hill, 1967.

Garber, R. S. "The Relationship of Psychiatry to Medicine." *Psychiatry Digest*, pp. 11-15, August 1969.

Gendzier, I. L. *Frantz Fanon: A Critical Study*. New York: Pantheon, 1973.

Glasscote, R. M.; Sanders, D.; Forstenzer, H. M.; and Foley, A. R. *The Community Mental Health Center: An Analysis of Existing Models*. Washington, D.C.: American Psychiatric Association, 1964.

―――; Sussex, J. N.; Cumming, E.; and Smith, L. H. *The Community Mental Health Center: An Interim Appraisal*. Washington, D.C.: American Psychiatric Association and National Association for Mental Health, 1969.

Glasser, W. *Schools Without Failure*. New York: Harper and Row, 1969.

Goffman, E. *Asylums: Essays on the Social Situation of Mental Patients and Other Inmates*. Garden City, N. Y.: Anchor Books, 1961.

Goldsmith, S. R., and Mandell, A. J. "The Dynamic Formulation—A Critique of Psychiatric Ritual." *American Journal of Psychiatry* 125(12):1738-1742, 1969.

Goldstein, A. S. *The Insanity Defense*. New Haven: Yale University Press, 1967.

Goldstein, J., and Katz, J. "Dangerousness and Mental Illness: Some Observations on the Decision to Release Persons Acquitted by Reason of Insanity." *Yale Law Journal* 70:225-239, 1960.

Goodman, P. *Growing Up Absurd: Problems of Youth in an Organized Society*. New York: Random House, 1962.

Green, R. "Homosexuality as a Mental Illness." *International Journal of Psychiatry* 10(1):77-98, 1972.

Grier, W. H., and Cobbs, P. M. *Black Rage*. New York: Basic Books, 1968.

Gursslin, O. R.; Hunt, R. G.; and Roach, J. L. "Social Class and the Mental Health Movement." In *Mental Health of the Poor*, edited by F. Riessman, J. Cohen, and A. Pearl. New York: The Free Press, 1964.

Guttmacher, M. "The Quest for a Test of Criminal Responsibility." *American Journal of Psychiatry* 11:428-433, 1954.

Guze, S. B.; Goodwin, D. W.; and Crane, J. B. "Criminality and Psychiatric Disorders." *Archives of General Psychiatry* 20:583-591, 1969.

Halleck, S. L. "American Psychiatry and the Criminal: A Historical Review." In *Current Psychiatric Therapies*, edited by J. H. Masserman. New York: Grune & Stratton, 1965.

―――. "Community Psychiatry: Some Troubling Questions." In *Community Psychiatry*, edited by L. M. Roberts, S. L. Halleck, M. B. Loeb. Garden City, N. Y.: Anchor Books, 1969.

―――. *The Politics of Therapy*. New York: Science House, 1971.

―――. *Psychiatry and the Dilemmas of Crime*. New York: Harper and Row, 1967.

――― and Bromberg, W. *Psychiatric Aspects of Criminology*. Springfield, Ill.: Charles C. Thomas, 1968.

Hamburg, D. A., ed. *Psychiatry as a Behavioral Science.* Englewood Cliffs, N. J.: Prentice-Hall, 1970.

Hamburg, D. A.; Bibring, G. L.; Fisher, C.; Stanton, A. H.; Wallerstein, R. S.; Weinstock, H. I.; and Haggard, E. "Report of Ad Hoc Committee on Central Fact-Gathering Data of the American Psychoanalytic Association." *Journal of the American Psychoanalytic Association* 15:841-861, 1967.

Hawkins, D., and Pauling, L., eds. *Orthomolecular Psychiatry.* San Francisco: Freeman, 1973.

Heller, J. *Catch-22.* New York: Simon and Schuster Inc., 1955.

Henry, W. E.; Sims, J. H.; and Spray, S. L. *The Fifth Profession.* San Francisco: Jossey-Bass, 1971.

Hilgard, E. R. *Theories of Learning.* 2d ed. New York: Appleton-Century-Crofts, 1956.

Hodge, P. "A Disturbed Life and a Violent Death." *Washington Post,* February 14, 1973. p. 1.

Hughes, H. S. *Consciousness and Society: The Reorientation of European Social Thought 1890-1930.* New York: Knopf, 1958.

Hunt, R. C., and Wiley, E. D. "Operation Baxstrom After One Year." *American Journal of Psychiatry* 124:974-978, 1968.

Huxley, A. *The Perennial Philosophy.* New York: Harper and Row, 1945.

"Incompetency Commitments Held Excessive by Harvard Study." *Psychiatric News,* May 2, 1973, pp. 20-21.

"Inmates' Records Doctored." *Medical World News,* May 5, 1972, pp. 17-18.

Jackson, B. "Reflections on DSM-II." *International Journal of Psychiatry* 7(6):385-392, 1969.

Jackson, D. "Action for Mental Illness—What Kind." *Stanford Medical Bulletin* 20:77-80, 1962.

Jahoda, M. *Current Concepts of Positive Mental Health.* Monograph Series No. 1. Joint Commission on Mental Illness and Health. New York: Basic Books, 1958.

Johannsen, W. J. "Attitudes Toward Mental Patients: A Review of Empirical Research." *Mental Hygiene* 53(2):218-228, 1969.

Jones, E. *The Life and Work of Sigmund Freud.* New York: Basic Books, 1955.

Jones, M. *The Therapeutic Community.* New York: Basic Books, 1953.

Jones, R. M. *Fantasy and Feeling in Education.* New York: New York University Press, 1968.

Kaplan, B., and Johnson, D. "The Social Meaning of Navaho Psychopathology and Psychotherapy." In *Magic, Faith, and Healing,* edited by A. Kiev. New York: The Free Press, 1964.

Kaplan, H. "Should Psychiatrists do Physical Examinations on Their Patients?" *Journal of the American Medical Association* 216(5):892, 1971.

Kaplan, L. *Mental Health and Human Relations in Education.* New York: Harper and Row, 1959.

Kardiner, A., and Ovesey, L. *Mark of Oppression.* New York: Meridian Books, 1962.

Katz, J.; Goldstein, J.; and Dershowitz, A. M. *Psychoanalysis, Psychiatry and Law.* New York: The Free Press, 1967.

Kaufman, M. R. "Psychiatry: Why 'Medical' or 'Social' Model?" *Archives of General Psychiatry* 17:347-360, 1967.

Kaufman, M. T. "Camp Offers a Haven for 1,000 of Bowery's Homeless." *New York Times*, December 18, 1972.

Keniston, K. "How Community Mental Health Stamped out the Riots (1968-78)." *Transaction* 5(8):21-29, 1968.

Kesey, K. *One Flew Over the Cuckoo's Nest.* New York: Viking Press, 1962.

Kiev, A., ed. *Magic, Faith, and Healing.* New York: The Free Press, 1964.

Kittrie, N. N. *The Right To Be Different: Deviance and Enforced Therapy.* Baltimore: Johns Hopkins Press, 1971.

Klein, H. E., and Temerlin, M. K. "Expert Testimony in Sanity Cases." *Journal of Nervous and Mental Disease* 149:435-438, 1969.

Klein, M. M., and Grossman, S. A. "Voting Competence and Mental Health." *American Journal of Psychiatry* 127(11):1562-1565, 1971.

Krasner, L. "Assessment of Token Economy Programs in Psychiatric Hospitals." In *The Role of Learning in Psychotherapy,* edited by R. Porter. Boston: Little, Brown, 1968.

Kubie, L. S. "Commitment." *Psychiatric News,* March 21, 1973, p. 2.

———. "Is Preventive Psychiatry Possible?" *Daedalus* 88:646-668, 1959.

———. "The Psychotherapeutic Ingredient in the Learning Process." *The Role of Learning in Psychotherapy,* edited by R. Porter. Boston: Little, Brown, 1968.

Kuhn, T. S. *The Structure of Scientific Revolutions.* Chicago: University of Chicago Press, 1962.

Laing, R. D. *The Politics of Experience.* New York: Pantheon, 1967.

Lamb, H. R., and Goertzel, V. "The Demise of the State Hospital—A Premature Obituary?" *Archives of General Psychiatry* 26:489-495, 1972.

Lasswell, H. D. "The Impact of Psychiatry Upon Jurisprudence." *Ohio State Law Review* 21:17-27, 1960.

Lazarus, R. S. *Psychological Stress and the Coping Process.* New York: McGraw-Hill, 1966.

Leedy, J. J. *Poetry Therapy: The Use of Poetry in the Treatment of Emotional Disorders.* Philadelphia: Lippincott, 1969.

Leifer, R. *In the Name of Mental Health: The Social Functions of Psychiatry.* New York: Science House, 1969.

Leighton, A. "Discussion." In *Transcultural Psychiatry* edited by A. V. S. deReuck and R. Porter. Boston: Little, Brown, 1965.

Lelyveld, J. "Obituary of Heroin Addict Who Died at 12." *The New York Times,* January 12, 1970, pp. 1 and 18.

Lemkau, P. V. "Prevention in Psychiatry." *American Journal of Public Health* 55(4):554-560, 1965.

Leuchter, H. J. "Are Schools To Be or Not To Be Mental Health Centers?" *American Journal of Psychiatry* 125(4):575-576, 1968.

Levine, A. "The Cold War Between Psychiatry and Psychology: A Psychiatrist's View." *Psychiatric Opinion* 4:5, 1967.

Levine, S. "Psychotherapy as Socialization." *International Journal of Psychiatry* 8(3):645-655, 1969.

Levy, L. "Operant Conditioning in Viet Nam. Letters to the Editor." *American Journal of Psychiatry* 124(8):1136, 1968.

Lindsey, R. "Sane or Insane? A Case Study of the TWA Hijacker." *New York Times,* January 18, 1973, pp. 43 and 49.

Linn, L. S. "State Hospital Environment and Rates of Patient Discharge." *Archives of General Psychiatry* 23(4):346-351, 1970.

Lipsitt, P. D.; Lelos, D.; and McGarry, A. L. "Competency for Trial: A Screening Instrument." *American Journal of Psychiatry* 128(1):105-109, 1971.

Livermore, J. M.; Malmquist, C. P.; and Meehl, P. E. "On the Justifications for Civil Commitment." *University of Pennsylvania Law Review* 117:75-96, 1968.

Lourie, N. V., and Walden, D. "The Lessons of Historical Reform Movements—The Racism-Mental Health Equation." *American Journal of Orthopsychiatry* 40(4):251, 1970.

Lyon, H. C. *Learning to Feel—Feeling to Learn.* Columbus: Merrill, 1971.

MacAndrew, C. "On the Notion that Certain Persons Who Are Given to Frequent Drunkenness Suffer from a Disease called Alcoholism." In *Changing Perspectives in Mental Illness,* edited by S. C. Plog and R. B. Edgerton. New York: Holt, Rinehart and Winston, 1969.

"Macing Mental Patients." *Medical World News,* March 6, 1970, pp. 18-19.

MacKenzie, J. P. "Nixon Details Anti-Crime Law Package." *Washington Post,* March 15, 1973, pp. 1 and 12.

Macleod, A., and Poland, P. "The Well-Being Clinic." *Social Work,* pp. 13-18, 1961.

Maisel, R. "Decision-Making in a Commitment Court." *Psychiatry* 33(3):352-361, 1970.

Mann, J. "Defendants Restricted on Insanity Plea." *Washington Post,* June 24, 1972, pp. 1 and 10.

Mariner, A. S. "A Critical Look at Professional Education in the Mental Health Field." *American Psychologist* 22:271-281, 1967.

Marmor, J. " 'Normal' and 'Deviant' Sexual Behavior." *Journal of the American Medical Association* 217(2):165-170, 1971.

Marzolf, S. S. "The Disease Concept in Psychology." *Psychological Review* 54:211-221, 1947.

Maslow, A. H. *Toward a Psychology of Being.* Princeton: Van Nostrand, 1962.

Matthews, A. R. "Mental Illness and the Criminal Law: Is Community Mental Health an Answer?" *American Journal of Public Health* 57(9):1571-1579, 1967.

May, R. "The Existential Approach." In *American Handbook of Psychiatry* Vol 2., edited by S. Arieti. New York: Basic Books, 1959, pp. 1348-1361.

McCabe, C. "On Looney Leaders." *San Francisco Chronicle,* September 30, 1969.

McCombs, P. A. "Free After 6 Years of Silence." *Washington Post,* June 22, 1972, pp. B1 and B4.

McGarry, A. L., and Greenblatt, M. "Conditional Voluntary Mental-Hospital Admission." *New England Journal of Medicine* 287(6):279-280, 1972.

McMorris, S. C. "Can We Punish for the Acts of Addiction?" *Bulletin on Narcotics* 22(3):43-48, 1970.

McNair, D. M.; Callahan, D. M.; and Lorr, M. "Therapist 'Type' and Patient Response to Psychotherapy." *Journal of Consulting Psychology* 26:425-429, 1962.

McNeil, J. N.; Llewellyn, C. E.; and McCollough, T. E. "Community Psychiatry and Ethics." *American Journal of Orthopsychiatry* 40(1):22-29, 1970.

Meerloo, J. A. M. "Hidden Suicide." In *Suicidal Behaviors,* edited by H. L. P. Resnik. Boston: Little, Brown, 1968.

Mehlman, B. "The Reliability of Psychiatric Diagnoses." *Journal of Abnormal and Social Psychology* Supplement, 47:2, 577-578, 1952.

Meltzer, H. Y. "Creatine Phosphokinase Activity and Clinical Symptomatology." *Archives of General Psychiatry* 29:589-593, 1973.

Mendel, W. M. "On the Abolition of the Psychiatric Hospital." In *Comprehensive Mental Health*, edited by C. M. Roberts, N. S. Greenfield, and M. H. Miller. Madison: University of Wisconsin Press, 1968.

———. "Responsibility in Health, Illness, and Treatment." *Archives of General Psychiatry* 18:697-705, 1968.

Menninger, K. *The Crime of Punishment.* New York: Viking Press, 1966.

———. "Sheer Verbal Mickey Mouse." *International Journal of Psychiatry* 7(6):415, 1969.

———. *The Vital Balance.* New York: Viking Press, 1963.

Mental Health Digest 1(10):56-57, 1969. Quoting in re Sealy, 218 So. 2nd 765, District Court of Appeal of Florida, First District, February 13, 1969.

"Mental Patients' Rights." *Civil Liberties,* September 1972, pp. 3-6.

Miller, D., and Schwartz, M. "County Lunacy Commission Hearings: Some Observations of Commitments to a State Mental Hospital." *Social Problems* 14:26-35, 1966.

Minde, K. K., and Werry, J. S. "Intensive Psychiatric Teacher Counseling in a Low Socioeconomic Area: A Controlled Evaluation." *American Journal of Orthopsychiatry* 39(4):595-608, 1969.

Mishler, E. G., and Scotch, N. A. "Sociocultural Factors in the Epidemiology of Schizophrenia." *Psychiatry* 26:315-351, 1963.

"Missouri Aims at Drug Assignment by Computer Setup." *Psychiatric News,* July 5, 1972.

"Modern Legal Test on Insanity Attacked by One of Its Drafters." *New York Times,* August 30, 1970.

Moore, R. "How Personality Difference of Students and Teachers Influence Students' Achievement." *People Watching* 2(1):31-34, 1972.

Morozov, G. V., and Kalashnik, I. M., eds. *Forensic Psychiatry.* White Plains, N. Y.: International Arts and Sciences Press, 1970. Originally published in Russian in 1967, translated by M. Vale.

Moustakas, C. E. *The Authentic Teacher: Sensitivity and Awareness in the Classroom.* Cambridge, Mass.: Doyle, 1966.

Mowrer, O. H. "Sin, the Lesser of Two Evils." *American Psychologist* 15:301-304, 1960.

National Institute of Mental Health. *Competency to Stand Trial and Mental Illness.* DHEW Publication No. 73-9105. Washington, D.C.: Government Printing Office, 1973.

Neill, A. S. *Summerhill.* New York: Hart, 1960.

Nelson, S., and Torrey, F. "The Religious Functions of Psychiatry." *American Journal of Orthopsychiatry* 43(3):362-367, 1973.

Nishimaru, S. "Mental Climate and Eastern Psychotherapy." *Transcultural Psychiatric Research* 2:24, April 1965.

Nunnally, J. C. *Popular Conceptions of Mental Health.* New York: Holt, Rinehart and Winston, 1961.

O'Connell, J. "The 'Crazy' Driver, the Car Maker, and Psychiatry. Letters to the Editor." *American Journal of Psychiatry* 124(8):1140-1142, 1968.

Ojemann, R. H. "Investigation on the Effects of Teaching an Understanding and Appreciation of Behavior Dynamics." In *Prevention of Mental Disorders in Children,* edited by G. Caplan. New York: Basic Books, 1961, pp. 378-397.

On Psychotherapy and Casework. New York: Group for the Advancement of Psychiatry, Publication No. 71, 1969.

Packer, H. L. *The Limits of Criminal Sanction.* Palo Alto: Stanford University Press, 1968.

Pande, S. K. "The Mystique of 'Western' Psychotherapy: An Eastern Interpretation." *Journal of Nervous and Mental Disease* 146(6):425-432, 1968.

Pasamanick, B.; Dinity, S.; and Lefton, M. "Psychiatric Orientation and Its Relation to Diagnosis and Treatment in a Mental Hospital." *American Journal of Psychiatry* 116(2):127-132, 1959.

Pearce, K. I. "A Comparison of Care Given by Family Practitioners and Psychiatrists in a Teaching Hospital Psychiatric Unit." *American Journal of Psychiatry* 127(6):835-840, 1970.

Pierce, C. M.; Mathis, J. L.; and Pishkin, V. "Basic Psychiatry in Twelve Hours." *Diseases of the Nervous System* 29:533-535, 1968.

Platt, A. M., and Diamond, B. L. "The Origins and Development of the 'Wild Beast' Concept of Mental Illness and Its Relation to Theories of Criminal Responsibility." *Journal of the History of the Behavioral Sciences* 1:4, 355-367, 1965.

Porter, R., ed. *The Role of Learning in Psychotherapy.* Boston: Little, Brown, 1968.

Poser, E. G. "The Effect of Therapists' Training on Group Therapeutic Outcome." *Journal of Consulting Psychology* 30(4):283-89, 1966.

Postman, N., and Weingartner, C. *The Soft Revolution.* New York: Dell, 1971.

———. *Teaching as a Subversive Activity.* New York: Delacorte, 1969.

Potter, H. C., and Stanton, G. T. "Money Management and Mental Health." *American Journal of Psychotherapy* 24(1):79-91, 1970.

"Preliminary Findings for the Psychiatric Inventory of Saint Elizabeth's Hospital." Prepared by the Hospital Staff. Washington, D.C.: May 31, 1970. Mimeographed.

Promotion of Mental Hygiene in the Primary and Secondary Schools: An Evaluation of Four Projects. Committee on Preventive Psychiatry. Report No. 18. New York: Group for the Advancement of Psychiatry, 1951.

Rabkin, J. G. "Opinions About Mental Illness: A Review of the Literature." *Psychological Bulletin* 77(3):153-171, 1972.

Rafferty, M. *On Education.* New York: Devin-Adair, 1968.

Rappeport, J. R. *The Clinical Evaluation of the Dangerousness of the Mentally Ill.* Springfield, Ill.: Charles C. Thomas, 1967.

——— and Lassen, G. "Dangerousness—Arrest Rate Comparisons of Discharged Patients and the General Population." *American Journal of Psychiatry* 121:776-783, 1965.

Redlich, F. C. "The Concept of Health in Psychiatry." In *Explorations in Social Psychiatry,* edited by A. H. Leighton; J. A. Clausen; and R. N. Wilson. New York: Basic Books, 1957.

——— and Freedman, D. X. *The Theory and Practice of Psychiatry.* New York: Basic Books, 1966.

——— and Pepper, M. "Are Social Psychiatry and Community Psychiatry Subspecialities of Psychiatry?" *American Journal of Psychiatry* 124(10):1343-1350, 1968.

Reider, N. "The Concept of Normality." *Psychoanalytic Quarterly* 19:43-51, 1950.

Reiff, R. "Social Intervention and the Problem of Psychological Analysis." *American Psychologist* 23:524-531, 1968.

Rhead, C.; Abrams, A.; Trosman, H.; and Margolis, P. "The Psychological Assessment of Police Candidates." *American Journal of Psychiatry* 124(11):1575-1580, 1968.

Riessman, F., and Miller, S. M. "Social Change Versus the 'Psychiatric World View.' " *American Journal of Orthopsychiatry* 34:29-38, 1964.

Roback, A. A. *A History of American Psychology.* New York: Collier Books, 1964.

Robitscher, J. "Courts, State Hospitals, and the Right to Treatment." *American Journal of Psychiatry* 129(3):298-304, 1972.

Roen, S. R. "The Behavioral Sciences in the Primary Grades." *American Psychologist* 20:430-432, 1965.

———. "Primary Prevention in the Classroom Through a Teaching Program in the Behavioral Sciences." In *Emergent Approaches to Mental Health Problems,* edited by E. L. Cowan; E. A. Gardner; and M. Zax. New York: Appleton-Century-Crofts, 1967.

Rogers, C. R. "The Characteristics of a Helping Relationship." *Personnel and Guidance Journal* 37:6-16, 1958.

———. *Client-Centered Therapy.* Boston: Houghton Mifflin, 1951.

———. "The Increasing Involvement of the Psychologist in Social Problems: Some Comments, Positive and Negative." *Journal of Applied Behavioral Science* 5(1):3, 1969.

———. "The Interpersonal Relationship in the Facilitation of Learning." In *The Helping Relationship Sourcebook,* edited by D. L. Avila; A. W. Combs; and W. W. Purkey. Boston: Allyn & Bacon, 1971.

———. *On Becoming a Person: A Therapist's View of Psychotherapy.* Boston: Houghton Mifflin, 1961.

Rogers, D. *Mental Hygiene in Elementary Education.* Boston: Houghton Mifflin, 1957.

Rogow, A. A. *The Psychiatrists.* New York: Putnam's, 1970.

Rosen, A. C. "Changes in the Perception of Mental Illness and Mental Health." *Perceptual and Motor Skills* 31(1):203-208, 1970.

Rosen, G. *Madness in Society: Chapters in the Historical Sociology of Mental Illness.* New York: Harper and Row, 1968.

Rosenhan, D. L. "On Being Sane in Insane Places." *Science* 179:250-258, January 19, 1973.

Rosenthal, R. "The Pygmalion Effect Lives." *Psychology Today* 7(4):56-63, 1973.

——— and Jacobson, L. *Pygmalion in the Classroom.* New York: Holt, Rinehart and Winston, 1968.

Ross, N. W. *Three Ways of Asian Wisdom.* New York: Simon & Schuster, 1966.

Ruesch, J., and Brodsky, C. M. "The Concept of Social Disability." *Archives of General Psychiatry* 19:394-403, 1968.

Ryan, W., ed. *Distress in the City.* Cleveland: Press of Case Western Reserve University, 1969.

Ryle, G. *The Concept of Mind.* Oxford: Hutchinson's University Press, 1948.

Sabshin, M. "Psychiatric Perspectives on Normality." *Archives of General Psychiatry* 17(3):258-264, 1967.
Sanford, N. "Education for Individual Development." *American Journal of Orthopsychiatry* 38(5):858-868, 1968.
Sarbin, T. R. "Anxiety: Reification of a Metaphor." *Archives of General Psychiatry* 10:630-638, 1964.
———. "Notes on the Transformation of Social Identity." In *Comprehensive Mental Health*, edited by L. M. Roberts; N. S. Greenfield; and M. H. Miller. Madison: University of Wisconsin Press, 1968.
———. "On the Futility of the Proposition that Some People be Labeled 'Mentally Ill.' " *Journal of Consulting Psychology* 31:447-453, 1967.
——— and Mancuso, J. C. "Paradigms and Moral Judgments: Improper Conduct Is Not Disease." *Journal of Consulting and Clinical Psychology* 39(1):6-8, 1972.
Satchell, M. "Retarded Are Easy Prey." *Washington Star-News,* August 7, 1973, p. 1.
Sauna, V. D. "Socio-Cultural Aspects of Psychotherapy and Treatment: A Review of the Literature." In *Progress in Clinical Psychology.* New York: Grune & Stratton, 1966.
Scheff, T. J. *Being Mentally Ill: A Sociological Theory.* Chicago: Aldine Publishing, 1966.
———. "The Societal Reaction to Deviance: Ascriptive Elements in the Psychiatric Screening of Mental Patients in a Midwestern State." *Social Problems* 11:401-413, 1964.
Schmidt, H. O., and Fonda, C. P. "The Reliability of Psychiatric Diagnosis, A New Look." *Journal of Abnormal and Social Psychology* 52(2):262-267, 1956.
Schur, E. M. *Our Criminal Society: The Social and Legal Sources of Crime in America.* Englewood Cliffs, N. J.: Prentice-Hall, 1969.
Schutz, W. C. *Joy: Expanding Human Awareness.* New York: Grove Press, 1967.
Schwartz, R. A. "The Role of Family Planning in the Primary Prevention of Mental Illness." *American Journal of Psychiatry* 125(12):1711-1718, 1969.
Schweitzer, A. *The Psychiatric Study of Jesus.* Boston: Beacon Press, 1948.
Seeley, J. R. *The Americanization of the Unconscious.* New York: International Science Press, 1967.
Serban, G. "Freudian Man Versus Existential Man." *Archives of General Psychiatry* 17:598-607, November 1967.
Shah, S. A. "Community Mental Health and the Criminal Justice System: Some Issues and Problems." *Mental Hygiene* 54(1):1-12, 1970.
———. "Crime and Mental Illness: Some Problems in Defining and Labeling Deviant Behavior." *Mental Hygiene* 53:21-33, 1969.
Shepard, M. *The Love Treatment: Sexual Intimacy Between Patients and Psychotherapists.* New York: Paperback Library, 1972.
Sherif, M., and Sherif, C. W. *Interdisciplinary Relationships in the Social Sciences.* Chicago: Aldine Publishing, 1969.
Shoben, E. J. "Some Observations on Psychotherapy and the Learning Process." In *Psychotherapy: Theory and Research,* edited by O. H. Mowrer. New York: Ronald Press, 1953.

———. "A Theoretical Approach to Psychotherapy as Personality Modification." *Harvard Educational Review* 23:128-142, 1953.

Silberman, C. E. *Crisis in the Classroom.* New York: Random House, 1970.

Sills, D. L. "Some Futures for the Social Sciences." In *Toward Century 21: Technology, Society, and Human Values,* edited by C. S. Wallia. New York: Basic Books, 1970.

Simon, R. J. "Mental Patients as Jurors." *Human Organization* 22(4):276-282, Winter 1963-1964.

The Social Responsibility of Psychiatrists: A Statement of Orientation. Report No. 13. Committee on Social Issues. New York: Group for the Advancement of Psychiatry, 1950.

Solomon, P. "The Burden of Responsibility in Suicide and Homicide." *Journal of the American Medical Association* 199:321-324, 1967.

Solzhenitsyn, I. *One Day in the Life of Ivan Denisovich.* New York: Praeger, 1963.

Soper, D. W., and Combs, A. W. "The Helping Relationship as Seen by Teachers and Therapists." *Journal of Consulting Psychology* 26:288, 1962.

Srole, L.; Langner, T. S.; Michael, S. T.; Opler, M. K.; and Rennie, T. A. C. *Mental Health in the Metropolis: The Midtown Manhattan Study.* New York: McGraw-Hill, 1962.

Steadman, H. J. "Follow-Up on Baxstrom Patients Returned to Hospitals for the Criminally Insane." *American Journal of Psychiatry* 130(3):317-319, 1973.

———. "The Psychiatrist as a Conservative Agent of Social Control." *Social Problems* 20(2):263-271, 1972.

Stiles, F. S. "Developing an Understanding of Human Behavior at the Elementary School Level." *Journal of Educational Research* 43:516-521, 1950.

Storrow, H. A. *Introduction to Scientific Psychiatry.* New York: Appleton-Century-Crofts, 1967.

Strupp, H. H. "Toward a Specification of Teaching and Learning in Psychotherapy." *Archives of General Psychiatry* 21:203-212, 1969.

Stunkard, A. "Some Interpersonal Aspects of an Oriental Religion." *Psychiatry* 14:419-431, 1951.

Suarez, J. "Psychiatry and the Criminal Law." *American Journal of Psychiatry* 129(3):293-297, 1972.

Sutich, A. J., and Vich, M. A. *Readings in Humanistic Psychology.* New York: The Free Press, 1969.

Swartz, J. "Role of the Psychiatrist. Letters to the Editor." *American Journal of Psychiatry* 124(9):1267, 1968.

Szasz, T. S. "Criminal Responsibility and Psychiatry." In *Legal and Criminal Psychology,* edited by H. Toch. New York: Holt, Rinehart and Winston, 1961.

———. *The Ethics of Psychoanalysis.* New York: Basic Books, 1965.

———. "Human Nature and Psychotherapy." *Comprehensive Psychiatry* 3:268-283, 1962.

———. *Law, Liberty, and Psychiatry.* New York: Macmillan, 1963.

———. *The Manufacture of Madness: A Comparative Study of the Inquisition and the Mental Health Movement.* New York: Dell, 1970.

———. *The Myth of Mental Illness.* New York: Harper and Row, 1961.

———. "Problems Facing Psychiatry: The Psychiatrist as Party to Conflict." In

Ethical Issues in Medicine: The Role of the Physician in Today's Society, edited by E. F. Torrey. Boston: Little, Brown, 1968.

———. "The Problem of Psychiatric Nosology." *American Journal of Psychiatry* 114(5):405-413, November 1957.

———. *Psychiatric Justice.* New York: Macmillan, 1965.

———. "Psychoanalysis and Suggestion." *Comprehensive Psychiatry* 4:271-280, 1963.

———. "Psychoanalysis and Taxation." *American Journal of Psychotherapy* 18:635-643, 1964.

———. "Psychoanalytic Treatment as Education." *Archives of General Psychiatry* 9(1):46-52, 1963.

———. "Voluntary Mental Hospitalization: An Unacknowledged Practice of Medical Fraud." *New England Journal of Medicine* 287(6):277-278, 1972.

———. "Whither Psychiatry?" *Social Research* 33(3):439-462, 1966.

——— and Alexander, G. J. "Law, Property and Psychiatry." *American Journal of Orthopsychiatry* 42(4):610-626, 1972.

——— and ———. "Mental Illness as Excuse for Civil Wrongs." *Journal of Nervous and Mental Disease* 147:113-123, 1968.

———; Knoff, W. F.; and Hollander, M. H. "The Doctor-Patient Relationship and Its Historical Context." *American Journal of Psychiatry* 115:522-528, 1958.

Tanay, E. "Psychiatric Study of Homicides." *American Journal of Psychiatry* 125(9):1252-1258, 1969.

Taylor, R. L., and Torrey, E. F. "The Pseudoregulation of American Psychiatry." *American Journal of Psychiatry* 129(6):658-662, 1972.

Temerlin, M. K. "Suggestion Effects in Psychiatric Diagnosis." *Journal of Nervous and Mental Disease* 147(4):349-353, 1968.

——— and Trousdale, W. W. "The Social Psychology of Clinical Diagnosis." *Psychotherapy: Theory, Research and Practice* 6(1):24-29, 1969.

Toffler, A. *Future Shock.* New York: Random House, 1970.

Torrey, E. F. "The Case for the Indigenous Therapist." *Archives of General Psychiatry* 20:365-373, 1969.

———. "Cheap Labor from Poor Nations." *American Journal of Psychiatry* 130:4, 428-433, 1973.

———. *The Mind Game: Witchdoctors and Psychiatrists.* New York: Emerson, 1972.

———. "Observations on Buddhism and Psychiatry in Thailand." *World Fellowship of Buddhists Bulletin* 7(1):16-19, 1970.

———. "Psychiatric Training: The SST of American Medicine." *Psychiatric Annals* 2(2):60-71, 1972.

——— and Peterson, M. R. "Slow and Latent Viruses in Schizophrenia." *Lancet* 2:22-24, July 7, 1973.

Tourney, G. "History of Biological Psychiatry in America." *American Journal of Psychiatry* 126(1):29-42, July 1969.

Train, D. "They Trained Us to Forget We Were Doctors." *Hospital Physician,* pp. 86-95, November 1968.

Truax, C. B., and Carkhuff, R. R. *Toward Effective Counseling and Psychotherapy: Training and Practice.* Chicago: Aldine Publishing, 1967.

Tucker, G. J.; Campion, E. W.; Kelleher, P. A.; and Silberfarb, P. M. "The Relationship of Subtle Neurologic Impairments to Disturbances of

Thinking." Read before the Second Congress of International College of Psychosomatic Medicine, Amsterdam, 1973.

Valentine, P. W. "Most at St. Elizabeth's Called Well Enough to Leave." *Washington Post,* August 11, 1971.

VanRheenen, F. J.; Torrey, E. F.; and Katchadourian, H. A. "Preventive Psychiatry: Group Work with Foreign Students." Presented at the Annual Meeting of the American Psychiatric Association, Washington, D.C., 1971.

Wallace, A. F. C. "Mental Illness, Biology, and Culture." In *Psychological Anthropology,* edited by F. L. K. Hsu. Homewood, Ill. Dorsey Press, 1961.

Wallerstein, R. S. "The Challenge of the Community Mental Health Movement to Psychoanalysis." *American Journal of Psychiatry* 124(8):1049-1056, February 1968.

Watts, A. W. *Psychotherapy East and West.* New York: Pantheon, 1961.

Weinstein, G., and Fantini, M. D. *Toward Humanistic Education: A Curriculum of Affect.* New York: Praeger, 1970.

Weintraub, W., and Aronson, H. "Is Classical Psychoanalysis a Dangerous Procedure?" *Journal of Nervous and Mental Disease* 149:224-228, 1969.

Werry, J. S. "Psychotherapy—A Medical Procedure?" *Canadian Psychiatric Association Journal* 10:278-282, 1965.

Williams, F. "Is There a Mental Hygiene?" *Psychoanalytic Quarterly* 1:113-120, 1932.

Wilson, J. *Education and the Concept of Mental Health.* London: Routledge and Kegan Paul, 1969.

Wiseman, F. "Psychiatry and Law: Use and Abuse of Psychiatry in a Murder Case." *American Journal of Psychiatry* 118:289-299, 1961.

Wittkower, E. D.; Cleghorn, J. M.; Lipowski, Z. J.; Peterfy, G.; and Solyom, L. "A Global Survey of Psychosomatic Medicine." *International Journal of Psychiatry* 7(1):499-516, 1969.

Woody, R. H. "Toward a Rationale for Psychobehavioral Therapy." *Archives of General Psychiatry* 19:197-204, 1968.

Wootton, B. *Social Science and Social Pathology.* London: George Allen and Unwin, 1959.

Wright, G. "Sirhan's Psyche Show." *San Francisco Examiner and Chronicle,* April 30, 1969.

Yalom, I. D. *The Theory and Practice of Group Psychotherapy.* New York: Basic Books, 1970.

Zilboorg, G., and Henry, G. W. *A History of Medical Psychology.* New York: Norton, 1941.

Zinberg, N. E. "Psychiatry: A Professional Dilemma." *Daedalus* 92(4):808-823, 1963.

Index

Some other books published by Penguin
are described on the following pages.

Allen Wheelis

THE MORALIST

The Moralist is Allen Wheelis's most powerful book, and its subject is nothing less than the survival of morals in a universe seemingly empty of everything but ignorance and maliciousness. In spite of this moral vacuum, Wheelis formulates a credo for modern man: "There is a path to follow, the course of which we cannot foresee, a plan of which we may have intimation but can never master. Whirl need not be king. Something draws us as by an invisible hand—not God, but the advancing edge of our being which goes before awareness." *The Moralist* is a meditation upon this "advancing edge," a confident yet illusionless look at the progress of man's awareness of others —a progress that is now humanity's only hope. Author of *The End of the Modern Age, The Desert,* and other books, Allen Wheelis is also a practicing psychoanalyst.

Malcolm B. Bowers, Jr., M.D.

RETREAT FROM SANITY
The Structure of Emerging Psychosis

This book is nothing less than a journey into the astonishing world of the psychotic. What is it like to experience psychosis? How does a developing psychotic perceive his environment? What clues tell him that he is sinking into madness? Dr. Malcolm B. Bowers, Jr., considers these questions through interviews with psychotic patients and through material written by the patients themselves—patients whose disturbances are associated with heterosexual rejection, psychosexual development, childbirth, or marital crisis. In this uniquely intimate way, readers of *Retreat from Sanity* meet a group of people who slipped out of reality and into a new dimension of distorted perceptions and bizarre thoughts. Malcolm B. Bowers, Jr., is Associate Professor of Psychiatry at Yale University School of Medicine.

Montague Ullman, M.D., and Stanley Krippner, Ph.D., with Alan Vaughan

DREAM TELEPATHY
Experiments in Nocturnal ESP

Here is the first totally reliable report on telepathic dreaming. Working from the hypothesis that ESP occurs more often in dreams than in consciousness, Dr. Montague Ullman and Dr. Stanley Krippner conducted experiments to determine whether a person acting as "agent" can transfer his thoughts to the mind of a sleeping "subject," thereby altering the subject's dreams. Recorded in this book are the intriguing results of their research: subjects' reactions, transcripts of dream sessions, accounts of unusual telepathic communication between participants, descriptions of experimental procedures, and a statistical summary. Appearing at a time when parapsychology is winning respect in both scientific and lay circles, *Dream Telepathy* bridges the gap between the rigorous standards of the scientists and the unproved claims of the psychics.

John G. Taylor

THE SHAPE OF MINDS TO COME

"A truly revolutionary development in man's understanding of his mind has occurred," writes John G. Taylor. "Already this new understanding of the mind has given birth to fantastic methods of controlling a man's behavior, or his feelings, or his intelligence." In this look at new knowledge about the workings and potential of the human mind, Taylor foresees a society able to wipe out aggressive and murderous instincts, to mold personality, to improve memory, and to regulate sexual appetites—all through startling advances in what is already being called mind mechanics. As Isaac Asimov has said, "This marvelously readable book takes you on a fantastic voyage and shows why the brains you and I possess may be the most wondrously complex structures in the universe." John G. Taylor is also the author of *Black Holes: The End of the Universe?*

RC
455.2
M4
T69

22, 515

CAMROSE LUTHERAN COLLEGE
LIBRARY